ADHD

Recent Titles in
Q&A Health Guides

Headaches: Your Questions Answered
Claudio Butticè

Healthy Technology Use: Your Questions Answered
Bernadette H. Schell

Autism: Your Questions Answered
Romeo Vitelli

ADHD

Your Questions Answered

Sarah Boslaugh

BLOOMSBURY ACADEMIC
NEW YORK • LONDON • OXFORD • NEW DELHI • SYDNEY

BLOOMSBURY ACADEMIC
Bloomsbury Publishing Inc
1385 Broadway, New York, NY 10018, USA
50 Bedford Square, London, WC1B 3DP, UK
29 Earlsfort Terrace, Dublin 2, Ireland

BLOOMSBURY, BLOOMSBURY ACADEMIC and the Diana logo are trademarks of
Bloomsbury Publishing Plc

First published in the United States of America 2024

Cover image © buritora/Adobe Stock

For legal purposes the Acknowledgments on p. xi constitute an
extension of this copyright page.

Bloomsbury Publishing Inc does not have any control over, or responsibility for,
any third-party websites referred to or in this book. All internet addresses given
in this book were correct at the time of going to press. The author and publisher
regret any inconvenience caused if addresses have changed or sites have ceased
to exist, but can accept no responsibility for any such changes.

This book discusses treatments (including types of medication and mental health
therapies), diagnostic tests for various symptoms and mental health disorders, and
organizations. The authors have made every effort to present accurate and up-to-date
information. However, the information in this book is not intended to recommend or
endorse particular treatments or organizations, or substitute for the care or medical
advice of a qualified health professional, or used to alter any medical therapy without
a medical doctor's advice. Specific situations may require specific therapeutic
approaches not included in this book. For those reasons, we recommend that readers
follow the advice of qualified health care professionals directly involved in their care.
Readers who suspect they may have specific medical problems should consult
a physician about any suggestions made in this book.

Library of Congress Cataloging-in-Publication Data
Names: Boslaugh, Sarah, author.
Title: ADHD : your questions answered / Sarah Boslaugh.
Other titles: Attention-deficit hyperactivity disorder : your questions answered
Description: New York : Bloomsbury Academic, 2024. |
Series: Q&A health guides | Includes index. | Audience: Grades 10-12
Identifiers: LCCN 2024005663 (print) | LCCN 2024005664 (ebook) |
ISBN 9781440880582 (hardback) | ISBN 9798765110447 (epub) |
ISBN 9781440880599 (ebook)
Subjects: LCSH: Attention-deficit hyperactivity disorder–Miscellanea.
Classification: LCC RJ506.H9 B67 2024 (print) |
LCC RJ506.H9 (ebook) | DDC 616.85/89–dc23/eng/20240305
LC record available at https://lccn.loc.gov/2024005663
LC ebook record available at https://lccn.loc.gov/2024005664

ISBN: HB: 978-1-4408-8058-2
         ePDF: 978-1-4408-8059-9
         eBook: 979-8-7651-1044-7

Series: Q&A Health Guides

Typeset by Integra Software Services Pvt. Ltd.
Printed and bound in the United States of America

To find out more about our authors and books visit www.bloomsbury.com
and sign up for our newsletters.

This book is dedicated to everyone affected by ADHD in the hopes that you may come to understand yourself better, access the resources you need, and live the life that you want.

Contents

Series Foreword

All of us have questions about our health. Is this normal? Should I be doing something differently? Whom should I talk to about my concerns? And our modern world is full of answers. Thanks to the internet, there's a wealth of information at our fingertips, from forums where people can share their personal experiences to Wikipedia articles to the full text of medical studies. But finding the right information can be an intimidating and difficult task—some sources are written at too high a level, others have been oversimplified, while still others are heavily biased or simply inaccurate.

Q&A Health Guides address the needs of readers who want accurate, concise answers to their health questions, authored by reputable and objective experts, and written in clear and easy-to-understand language. This series focuses on the topics that matter most to young adult readers, including various aspects of physical and emotional well-being as well as other components of a healthy lifestyle. These guides will also serve as a valuable tool for parents, school counselors, and others who may need to answer teens' health questions.

All books in the series follow the same format to make finding information quick and easy. Each volume begins with an essay on health literacy and why it is so important when it comes to gathering and evaluating health information. Next, the top five myths and misconceptions that surround the topic are dispelled. The heart of each guide is a collection of questions and answers, organized thematically. A selection of five case studies provides real-world examples to illuminate key concepts. Rounding out each volume are a directory of resources, glossary, and index.

It is our hope that the books in this series will not only provide valuable information but will also help guide readers toward a lifetime of healthy decision-making.

Acknowledgments

There may be only one author credited for this book, but it draws on the works of many eminent clinicians and researchers who have contributed to our understanding of ADHD specifically and neurodiversity more generally. Beyond that, I owe a debt to all my professors at the University of Nebraska and the Graduate Center of the City University of New York for teaching me the research, writing, and analytic skills that have made my career possible.

This book would not exist without the insights and feedback provided by Maxine Taylor, my editor at ABC-CLIO, who expertly shepherded me through the stages of writing it. Even more crucially, it would not exist without the professional services provided by the Community Psychological Service of the University of Missouri, St. Louis, in particular those of Julia Sager, BS, and John Nanney, Ph.D. They diagnosed me, at the age of 62, with ADHD, a diagnosis that explained many things about my life and set me on a journey of self-discovery that has not yet concluded.

Introduction

ADHD (Attention-Deficit/Hyperactivity Disorder) is one of the most common neurodevelopmental disorders of childhood, with some national surveys finding that more than 10 percent of school-age children in the United States have ADHD. While early researchers believed ADHD occurred only among children, and primarily among boys, today we know that people of any gender, age, race, or ethnic group can have ADHD. Yet many people do not understand ADHD and may hold mistaken beliefs about it, sometimes even doubting that it is a real condition. This book, while not a substitute for professional advice, is intended to help educate readers about ADHD and to point them to reliable resources from which they can seek further help.

ADHD is recognized today as a psychiatric condition that can affect many aspects of a person's life, from performing well in school and at work to forming healthy and lasting social, romantic, and familial relationships. The definition of ADHD and the diagnostic criteria used to diagnose it have evolved over the years—two facts it shares with many other psychiatric conditions. According to the fifth edition of the *Diagnostic and Statistical Manual* (*DSM-5*) of the American Psychiatric Association, which is the standard authority used by health professionals to define and diagnose psychiatric disorders in the United States, there are three subtypes of ADHD: predominantly inattentive, predominantly hyperactive, and combined type (both inattentive and hyperactive).

Examples of inattentive behaviors include making careless mistakes in schoolwork or on the job, allowing your attention to drift away when someone is speaking to you, failing to follow clear directions or to complete tasks in an appropriate sequence, and frequently forgetting or losing things such as your cellphone, keys, or glasses. Examples of hyperactive behaviors include fidgeting, constantly feeling jumpy or restless, being unable to work or play quietly, talking excessively and without regard to social norms, and failing to wait one's turn in a game or an activity. Combined type ADHD simply means that both inattentive and hyperactive behaviors are present.

Many people with ADHD struggle with executive functions, skills that allow them to control and coordinate their other cognitive abilities and behaviors. The executive functions perform tasks analogous to that of a person holding an executive job in a business context: the executive is tasked with making long-term plans and monitoring the company's progress toward them, while lower-level employees carry out the necessary tasks to fulfill those plans and respond to feedback from the executive. As a child matures into an adult, they are expected to develop improved executive functioning so that they can take on more responsibility for planning their activities and can carry out long-term projects, but many people with ADHD find it difficult to meet these expectations.

Three main executive functions have been identified: working memory, cognitive flexibility, and inhibition control. Working memory refers to the information held in the "front of your mind" that is easily accessible while you perform a specific cognitive task, for instance, remembering a telephone number long enough to dial it. Cognitive flexibility means the ability to shift your mind from one topic to another, or to switch between approaches to a topic or situation when it is beneficial to do so, for instance, trying multiple ways to solve a math problem until you come up with one that works. Inhibition control is the ability to manage and control one's thoughts, emotions, and behaviors, in order to complete tasks and behave in a socially acceptable manner.

Because many people remain unaware of ADHD or hold false beliefs about it, people with ADHD may not be identified and thus remain unable to access the support and treatment they need. Symptoms of ADHD can easily be misinterpreted as misbehavior, laziness, or lack of desire, and undiagnosed and untreated ADHD can make it difficult for a person to function well in school, in a career, and in personal relationships. Fortunately, many types of treatment are available today for ADHD, and appropriate treatment and support can help the person affected understand themselves better and succeed in whatever path they have chosen in life.

I hope everyone who reads this book comes away with a better understanding of ADHD and how it can affect a person's functioning. I also hope it helps to dispel prejudices and misinformation and helps people understand that everyone's mind works differently and that neurodiversity can be a wonderful thing. Finally, as a person who was diagnosed with ADHD in adulthood, I also hope it helps people who think they might have ADHD, but have never been formally evaluated for it, to seek out the best evaluation and treatment available.

Guide to Health Literacy

On her 13th birthday, Samantha was diagnosed with type 2 diabetes. She consulted her mom and her aunt, both of whom also have type 2 diabetes, and decided to go with their strategy of managing diabetes by taking insulin. As a result of participating in an after-school program at her middle school that focused on health literacy, she learned that she can help manage the level of glucose in her bloodstream by counting her carbohydrate intake, following a diabetic diet, and exercising regularly. But, what exactly should she do? How does she keep track of her carbohydrate intake? What is a diabetic diet? How long should she exercise and what type of exercise should she do? Samantha is a visual learner, so she turned to her favorite source of media, YouTube, to answer these questions. She found videos from individuals around the world sharing their experiences and tips, doctors (or at least people who have "Dr." in their YouTube channel names), government agencies such as the National Institutes of Health, and even video clips from cat lovers who have cats with diabetes. With guidance from the librarian and the health and science teachers at her school, she assessed the credibility of the information in these videos and even compared their suggestions to some of the print resources that she was able to find at her school library. Now, she knows exactly how to count her carbohydrate level, how to prepare and follow a diabetic diet, and how much (and what) exercise is needed daily. She intends to share her findings with her mom and her aunt, and now she wants to create a chart that summarizes what she has learned that she can share with her doctor.

Samantha's experience is not unique. She represents a shift in our society; an individual no longer views himself or herself as a passive recipient of medical care but as an active mediator of his or her own health. However, in this era when any individual can post his or her opinions and experiences with a particular health condition online with just a few clicks or publish a memoir, it is vital that people know how to assess the credibility of health information. Gone are the days when "publishing" health information required intense vetting. The health information landscape is highly saturated, and people have innumerable sources where they can find information about practically any health topic.

The sources (whether print, online, or a person) that an individual consults for health information are crucial because the accuracy and trustworthiness of the information can potentially affect his or her overall health. The ability to find, select, assess, and use health information constitutes a type of literacy—health literacy—that everyone must possess.

The Definition and Phases of Health Literacy

One of the most popular definitions for health literacy comes from Ratzan and Parker (2000), who describe health literacy as "the degree to which individuals have the capacity to obtain, process, and understand basic health information and services needed to make appropriate health decisions." Recent research has extrapolated health literacy into health literacy bits, further shedding light on the multiple phases and literacy practices that are embedded within the multifaceted concept of health literacy. Although this research has focused primarily on online health information seeking, these health literacy bits are needed to successfully navigate both print and online sources. There are six phases of health information seeking: (1) Information Need Identification and Question Formulation, (2) Information Search, (3) Information Comprehension, (4) Information Assessment, (5) Information Management, and (6) Information Use.

The first phase is the *information need identification and question formulation phase*. In this phase, one needs to be able to develop and refine a range of questions to frame one's search and understand relevant health terms. In the second phase, *information search*, one has to possess appropriate searching skills, such as using proper keywords and correct spelling in search terms, especially when using search engines and databases. It is also crucial to understand how search engines work (i.e., how search results are derived, what the order of the search results means, how to use the snippets that are provided in the search results list to select websites, and how to determine which listings are ads on a search engine results page). One also has to limit reliance on surface characteristics, such as the design of a website or a book (a website or book that appears to have a lot of information or looks aesthetically pleasant does not necessarily mean it has good information) and language used (a website or book that utilizes jargon, the keywords that one used to conduct the search, or the word "information" does not necessarily indicate it will have good information). The next phase is *information comprehension*, whereby one needs to have the ability to read, comprehend, and recall the information (including textual, numerical, and visual content) one has located from the books and/or online resources.

To assess the credibility of health information (*information assessment* phase), one needs to be able to evaluate information for accuracy, evaluate how current the information is (e.g., when a website was last updated or when a book was published), and evaluate the creators of the source— for example, examine site sponsors or type of sites (.com, .gov, .edu, or .org) or the author of a book (e.g., practicing doctor, a celebrity doctor, a patient of a specific disease) to determine the believability of the person/ organization providing the information. Such credibility perceptions tend to become generalized, so they must be frequently reexamined (e.g., the belief that a specific news agency always has credible health information needs continuous vetting). One also needs to evaluate the credibility of the medium (e.g., television, internet, radio, social media, and book) and evaluate—not just accept without questioning—others' claims regarding the validity of a site, book, or other specific source of information. At this stage, one has to "make sense of information gathered from diverse sources by identifying misconceptions, main and supporting ideas, conflicting information, point of view, and biases" (American Association of School Librarians [AASL], 2009, p. 13) and conclude which sources/information are valid and accurate by using conscious strategies rather than simply using intuitive judgments or "rules of thumb." This phase is the most challenging segment of health information seeking and serves as a determinant of success (or lack thereof) in the information-seeking process. The following section on Sources of Health Information further explains this phase.

The fifth phase is *information management*, whereby one has to organize information that has been gathered in some manner to ensure easy retrieval and use in the future. The last phase is *information use*, in which one will synthesize information found across various resources, draw conclusions, and locate the answer to his or her original question and/or the content that fulfills the information need. This phase also often involves implementation, such as using the information to solve a health problem; make health-related decisions; identify and engage in behaviors that will help a person to avoid health risks; share the health information found with family members and friends who may benefit from it; and advocate more broadly for personal, family, or community health.

The Importance of Health Literacy

The conception of health has moved from a passive view (someone is either well or ill) to one that is more active and process based (someone is working toward preventing or managing disease). Hence, the dominant focus has shifted from doctors and treatments to patients and prevention, resulting in the need to strengthen our ability and confidence (as patients and consumers of health care) to look for, assess, understand, manage, share, adapt, and use health-related information. An individual's health literacy level has been found to predict his or her health status better than age, race, educational attainment, employment status, and income level (National Network of Libraries of Medicine, 2013). Greater health literacy also enables individuals to better communicate with health care providers such as doctors, nutritionists, and therapists, as they can pose more relevant, informed, and useful questions to health care providers. Another added advantage of greater health literacy is better information-seeking skills, not only for health but also in other domains, such as completing assignments for school.

Sources of Health Information: The Good, the Bad, and the In-Between

For generations, doctors, nurses, nutritionists, health coaches, and other health professionals have been the trusted sources of health information. Additionally, researchers have found that young adults, when they have health-related questions, typically turn to a family member who has had firsthand experience with a health condition because of their family member's close proximity and because of their past experience with, and trust in, this individual. Expertise should be a core consideration when consulting a person, website, or book for health information. The credentials and background of the person or author and conflicting interests of the author (and his or her organization) must be checked and validated to ensure the likely credibility of the health information they are conveying. While books often have implied credibility because of the peer-review process involved, self-publishing has challenged this credibility, so qualifications of book authors should also be verified. When it comes to health information, currency of the source must also be examined. When examining health information/studies presented, pay attention to the exhaustiveness of research methods utilized to offer recommendations or conclusions. Small and nondiverse sample size is often—but not always—an indication of reduced credibility. Another potential issue to watch for is studies that confuse correlation with causation. Information seekers must also pay attention to the sponsors of the research studies. For example, if a study is sponsored by manufacturers of drug Y and the study recommends that drug Y is the best treatment to manage or cure a disease, this may indicate a lack of objectivity on the part of the researchers.

The internet is rapidly becoming one of the main sources of health information. Online forums, news agencies, personal blogs, social media sites, pharmacy sites, and celebrity "doctors" are all offering medical and health information targeted to various types of people in regard to all types of diseases and symptoms. There are professional journalists, citizen journalists, hoaxers, and people paid to write fake health news on various sites that may appear to have a legitimate domain name and may even have authors who claim to have professional credentials, such as an MD. All these sites *may* offer useful information or information that appears to be useful and relevant; however, much of the information may be debatable and may fall into gray areas that require readers to discern credibility, reliability, and biases.

While broad recognition and acceptance of certain media, institutions, and people often serve as the most popular determining factors to assess credibility of health information among young people, keep in mind that there are legitimate internet sites, databases, and books that publish health information and serve as sources of health information for doctors, other health sites, and members of the public. For example, MedlinePlus (https://medlineplus.gov) has trusted sources on over 975 diseases and conditions and presents the information in easy-to-understand language.

The chart here presents factors to consider when assessing credibility of health information. However, keep in mind that these factors function only as a guide and require continuous updating to keep abreast with the changes in the landscape of health information, information sources, and technologies.

The chart can serve as a guide; however, approaching a librarian about how one can go about assessing the credibility of both print and online health information is far more effective than using generic checklist-type tools. While librarians are not health experts, they can apply and teach patrons strategies to determine the credibility of health information.

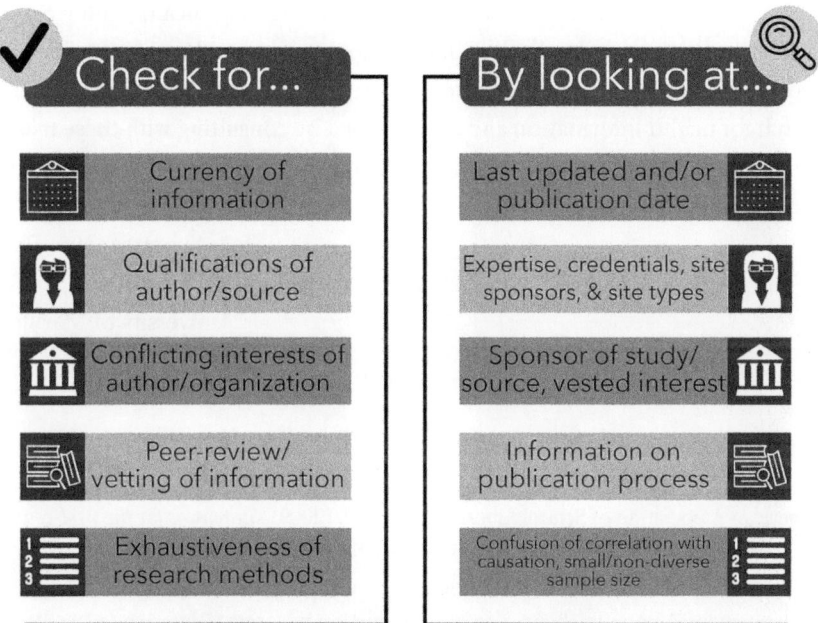

All images from flaticon.com

With the prevalence of fake sites and fake resources that appear to be legitimate, it is important to use the following health information assessment tips to verify health information that one has obtained (St. Jean et al., 2015, p. 151):

- **Don't assume you are right**: Even when you feel very sure about an answer, keep in mind that the answer may not be correct, and it is important to conduct (further) searches to validate the information.
- **Don't assume you are wrong**: You may actually have correct information, even if the information you encounter does not match—that is, you may be right and the resources that you have found may contain false information.
- **Take an open approach**: Maintain a critical stance by not including your preexisting beliefs as keywords (or letting them influence your choice of keywords) in a search, as this may influence what it is possible to find out.
- **Verify, verify, and verify**: Information found, especially on the internet, needs to be validated, no matter how the information appears on the site (i.e., regardless of the appearance of the site or the quantity of information that is included).

Health literacy comes with experience navigating health information. Professional sources of health information, such as doctors, health care providers, and health databases, are still the best, but one also has the power to search for health information and then verify it by consulting with these trusted sources and by using the health information assessment tips and guide shared previously.

Mega Subramaniam, Ph.D.
Associate Professor, College of Information Studies,
University of Maryland

References and Further Reading

American Association of School Librarians (AASL). (2009). *Standards for the 21st-century learner in action.* Chicago, IL: American Association of School Librarians.

Hilligoss, B., & Rieh, S.-Y. (2008). "Developing a unifying framework of credibility assessment: Construct, heuristics, and interaction in context." *Information Processing & Management,* 44(4), 1467–84.

Kuhlthau, C. C. (1988). "Developing a model of the library search process: Cognitive and affective aspects." *Reference Quarterly,* 28(2), 232–42.

National Network of Libraries of Medicine (NNLM). (2013). *Health literacy.* Bethesda, MD: National Network of Libraries of Medicine. Retrieved from nnlm.gov/outreach/consumer/hlthlit.html

Ratzan, S. C., & Parker, R. M. (2000). "Introduction." In C. R. Selden, M. Zorn, S. C. Ratzan, & R. M. Parker (Eds.), *National Library of Medicine current bibliographies in medicine: Health literacy.* NLM Pub. No. CBM 2000–1. Bethesda, MD: National Institutes of Health, U.S. Department of Health and Human Services.

St. Jean, B., Taylor, N. G., Kodama, C., & Subramaniam, M. (February 2017). "Assessing the health information source perceptions of tweens using card-sorting exercises." *Journal of Information Science.* Retrieved from http://journals.sagepub.com/doi/abs/10.1177/0165551516687728

St. Jean, B., Subramaniam, M., Taylor, N. G., Follman, R., Kodama, C., & Casciotti, D. (2015). "The influence of positive hypothesis testing on youths' online health-related information seeking." *New Library World,* 116(3/4), 136–54.

Subramaniam, M., St. Jean, B., Taylor, N. G., Kodama, C., Follman, R., & Casciotti, D. (2015). "Bit by bit: Using design-based research to improve the health literacy of adolescents." *JMIR Research Protocols,* 4(2), paper e62. Retrieved from http://www.ncbi.nlm.nih.gov/pmc/articles/PMC4464334/

Valenza, J. (November 26, 2016). Truth, truthiness, and triangulation: A news literacy toolkit for a "post-truth" world [Web log]. Retrieved from http://blogs.slj.com/neverendingsearch/2016/11/26/truth-truthiness-triangulation-and-the-librarian-way-a-news-literacy-toolkit-for-a-post-truth-world/

Common Misconceptions about ADHD

1. Only children can have ADHD

While it was once believed that ADHD occurred only during childhood, today we know this is not the case. Children with ADHD do not simply "grow out" of it as they mature, although they may learn ways to control their condition and cope with its symptoms so it seems to an observer that they are no longer affected by ADHD. In addition, some adults today are being diagnosed with ADHD despite never having received that diagnosis in childhood. For many years, the belief that only children could have ADHD, combined with diagnostic criteria based on studies of children, acted as a sort of self-fulfilling prophecy: it seemed that no adults had ADHD because medical and psychological professionals were taught that it was a condition of childhood, and the diagnostic criteria for ADHD was based on observations of children. For more about adult ADHD, see Questions 1, 3, and 12.

2. Only boys can have ADHD

For many years ADHD was believed to occur only in boys, and it remains true today that more boys and men are diagnosed with ADHD than are girls and women. However, today we know that ADHD can occur in people of any gender, and clinicians are becoming more aware of the differences in how ADHD can present in males and females, and diagnostic criteria may be updated in the future so that the discrepancy lessens or disappears. In general, males with ADHD are more likely to display hyperactive and impulsive symptoms, while females are more likely to experience inattentive symptoms, and are also more likely to report experiencing depression and anxiety than are boys or non-ADHD female controls. It may also be the case that the hyperactive and impulsive symptoms of ADHD, which are more common among boys, are likely to disrupt a school or workplace environment, and thus the individual causing the disruption may be referred for evaluation. In contrast, the quieter symptoms such as withdrawing from a social environment, which are more typical of girls, may be overlooked because they are not causing an immediate problem. For more about ADHD in girls and women, see Questions 2, 3, and 11.

3. ADHD can only be controlled through medication

Some people with ADHD do take medication for their condition, but this practice is by no means universal. Decisions about medication and other treatments should always be based on medical advice that takes into account the needs and desires of the individual patient, and many types of treatments for ADHD are available today besides drug therapy, including behavior management, cognitive-behavioral therapy, and practices such as yoga. Sometimes people find that a combination of treatments works best for them, and the goal of any plan of treatment should be to find what works best for the individual patient. Fear of being prescribed drugs should never be a reason to avoid professional advice, and the patient (and/or the parents in the case of children) should not be afraid to ask about alternatives. For more about non drug treatments for ADHD, see Questions 26, 27, and 28.

4. People with ADHD can't succeed in school, work, or life

People with ADHD have a special set of challenges to face, but that doesn't mean that they can't be successful in whatever they choose to do. The key is to get a correct diagnosis and to find a treatment or combination of treatments that works for the individual, as well as appropriate guidance to help the person with ADHD understand their condition and ways that they can help themselves succeed in life. All the burden should not be placed on the individual with ADHD, however: there are many things that family members can do to help, particularly if the person with ADHD is a child. Schools can make adjustments to help students with ADHD succeed, and the same is true of the workplaces. Sometimes small adjustments can make a big difference, and in both schools and workplaces in the United States, people with ADHD are entitled to reasonable accommodations if they ask for them. In addition, some people with ADHD have come to regard it as a sort of superpower that most people don't have. For instance, hyperfocus may give people an advantage when working for long periods on exacting scientific problems. For more about success for people with ADHD, see Questions 36, 37, 39, 40, and 41.

5. People with ADHD just need to try harder

Many people with ADHD share one experience that they wish they didn't—having their condition dismissed as nonexistent and their difficulties in behaving in societally expected ways as due to character flaws or lack of effort. Medical and psychological professionals today agree that ADHD is a real condition that is diagnosed using specific criteria based on observation, interviews, and psychological testing. Unfortunately, even today some people do believe that if people with ADHD just tried harder, their difficulties would disappear. To a person with ADHD, that sounds like telling a deaf person they could hear if they just applied themselves to the task. Such remarks are based in ignorance and/or prejudice, and while it's not the job of every person with ADHD to educate the general public on their condition, for those who feel up to the task, there's no harm in being armed with some relevant facts. For more information about educating people about the reality of ADHD, see Questions 5, 9, and 45.

Questions and Answers

1

The Basics

1. What is ADHD, and are there different types?

ADHD stands for Attention Deficit Hyperactivity Disorder, a psychiatric condition that can make it more difficult for a person to function well in school, at work, and in social and familial relationships. While every person's experience of ADHD is unique, common symptoms of ADHD include inattentiveness, impulsivity, and hyperactivity. People with ADHD often have difficulty with executive functioning, a set of skills that help people plan for the future; set goals for themselves; and monitor their progress toward their goals. Executive function skills become increasingly important as a student progresses from elementary school through high school and college, as assignments get longer and students are expected to play a greater role in managing their own time, it is important for anyone having difficulty with these skills to receive help as soon as problems arise.

One tricky thing about ADHD is that the behaviors which define it are commonly seen in many people, and it can be a judgment call as to when such behaviors become a problem that requires a response. Who among us has not found their mind wandering during a boring lecture, failed to complete an assignment exactly as directed, or found themselves blurting something out instead of waiting for an appropriate moment to speak? The difference is that for most people, these are occasional lapses that don't cause serious difficulty to their ability to thrive. For a person with ADHD, on the other hand, such troubling symptoms tend to occur more frequently, to be more severe, and may interfere with their ability to succeed in school or at work and to have normal relationships with other people.

ADHD was first identified in children and is still most often diagnosed in childhood, because the symptoms of ADHD may make it difficult for a child to function in a school context. It's important to spot ADHD symptoms in children and follow up as necessary, because children with undiagnosed ADHD may fall behind their peers and their actions be labeled as misbehavior or lack of ability, while they may doubt their own intelligence and ability to succeed. The purpose of having someone evaluated for ADHD is not to pin a label on them but to help them understand themselves and to create conditions so they can succeed in life.

Although it's more common to get an ADHD diagnosis in childhood, some people are not diagnosed until adulthood. A number of different symptoms can be used to diagnose ADHD, and not all need be present in one individual. For instance, despite the name of this condition, not all people with ADHD exhibit hyperactive behavior. As with any psychiatric evaluation, a person's symptoms and behaviors are always evaluated in terms of what is considered normal or expected for their age, maturity level, and culture, and in the relevant context (e.g., considering that some behaviors may be completely normal and acceptable on the playground or at home but not appropriate to a school classroom). An ADHD diagnosis also requires ruling out any other possible explanations for the observed behaviors, including other clinical disorders such as depression or anxiety, learning disorders such as dyslexia, impairment of hearing or vision, and substance abuse.

The definition of ADHD and the criteria use to diagnose it have changed over the years, as more researchers have studied ADHD and medical professionals have come to understand more about this condition. Currently the fifth edition of the *Diagnostic and Statistical Manual* (*DSM-5*) of the American Psychiatric Association, which is the standard authority used by health professionals to define and diagnose psychiatric disorders in the United States, defines three subtypes of ADHD:

1. Predominantly inattentive
2. Predominantly hyperactive
3. Combined type (both inattentive and hyperactive)

Examples of inattentive behaviors include making careless mistakes in schoolwork or on the job, when lack of knowledge is not the issue; letting your mind drift away from the subject at hand when reading or attending a class lecture; failing to pay attention when someone is speaking to you; failing to follow clear directions or to complete tasks in an appropriate sequence; frequently forgetting or losing things such as your cellphone, keys, or glasses; starting a project with great enthusiasm, then losing focus and getting sidetracked so it is never completed; and missing deadlines for an important project you had every intent to complete. Students displaying inattentive behavior may be scolded, causing them to experience shame or guilt, and the student may come to decide that "I'm just not smart" or "school is not for me" and set expectations for themselves lower than their abilities merit. Adults displaying these behaviors may be judged as unreliable or not taking their job duties seriously, and may internalize those judgments and give up on themselves.

Examples of hyperactive behaviors include fidgeting or constantly feeling jumpy or restless; jumping out of one's seat without permission and running around the room; being unable to work or play quietly; talking excessively and without regard to social norms; speaking out of turn and interrupting others; and failing to wait one's turn in a game or activity. A teacher unaware of the symptoms of ADHD may interpret these actions as misbehavior, particularly if they interfere with the normal functioning of the classroom, while peers may simply not want to be friends with someone who behaves unpredictably or violates basic social norms like taking turns in a game. Hyperactive behaviors may also be interpreted as threatening, particularly if the person displaying them is large, and may result in school security or law enforcement being summoned to subdue disruptive behaviors or remove the person from the classroom. A student displaying hyperactive behaviors may be frustrated with themselves and wish to conform to expectations, or may embrace the label placed on them, concentrating more on disrupting the classroom or social environment than in working within it. Combined type ADHD simply means that both inattentive and hyperactive behaviors are present.

2. How prevalent is ADHD, and is it becoming more common?

ADHD is a common childhood disorder, and the number of people diagnosed with it has been increasing for the past several decades. In the United States, data collected by the National Health Interview Survey found that in 1997–8 6.1 percent of children aged 4–17 had been identified as having ADHD, while in 2015–16, 10.2 percent had been identified as having ADHD. This is a 67.2 percent increase, meaning that almost 2/3 more children and adolescents were diagnosed with ADHD in 2015–16 than in 1997–8. ADHD diagnoses have also increased over these years in both children and adolescents, in both boys and girls, and in all racial groups studied.

ADHD in adults has been studied less than ADHD in children. This is due in part to the fact that ADHD was originally thought to be exclusively a childhood disorder, so a first diagnosis in adulthood was not possible. Although diagnostic standards have changed to include adults, it's still less common for adults to be evaluated for ADHD, as compared to children. For these reasons, it's more difficult to determine how many adults in the United States have ADHD or to see how that number has changed over time. One survey estimated that 4.4 percent of US adults aged 18–44 have ADHD, and that 8.1 percent of people in that age group have received an ADHD diagnosis at some point in their lives (in either childhood or adulthood).

Determining the global prevalence of ADHD is more complicated, because of varying cultural norms and expectations, as well as differences in the availability of psychiatric care across countries. However, a 2015 meta-analysis of 175 studies by Rae Thomas and colleagues estimated that, globally, 7.2 percent of children age 17 and under had ADHD. As in the United States, most countries have historically placed more emphasis on diagnosing ADHD in children rather than adults, so less data is available on adult ADHD globally. However, a study by John Fayyad and colleagues involving over 11,000 adults from 10 countries in the Americas, Europe, and the Middle East estimated that 3.4 percent of adults globally have ADHD.

There are many possible explanations for the observable fact that more people are being diagnosed with ADHD today than in the past, and the best explanation may lie in a combination of these factors. The simplest possibility is that more people have this condition than in the past, so the increase in diagnoses accurately reflects an increase in the occurrence of ADHD. Another possible explanation is that increased awareness of ADHD and the importance of evaluating and treating it from an early age have motivated more parents to take their children in for evaluation, more school systems to invest resources in identifying and helping children with ADHD, and more insurance companies to pay for psychiatric evaluations and other services for people with ADHD. This explanation may be particularly relevant for adult ADHD, since until recently ADHD was considered a condition that only occurred in childhood, and one that a child would grow out of in time. Given the current awareness that ADHD may persist over a person's lifetime, an adult with symptoms suggesting ADHD now has the possibility of seeking and getting a diagnosis, which would not have been possible in the past.

Another possible explanation is that the stigma of ADHD has declined and more effective treatments are available to help people with ADHD, so that more people are willing to be evaluated, accept a diagnosis of ADHD, and report this diagnosis on surveys. A fourth and related possibility is that the availability of educational accommodations for ADHD, such as increased time to take exams, may be encouraging some students and parents to be more willing to seek and accept a diagnosis of ADHD. In fact, it has been suggested that some parents and/or children are gaming the system to get an ADHD diagnosis (for instance, by doctor shopping until they find one willing to provide the diagnosis) and get access to accommodations that they believe will give them an advantage, but it's difficult to say how often this occurs, if at all. Most importantly, the possibility of incorrect diagnosis does not justify calling any individual's diagnosis or accommodations into question without hard evidence to suggest a mistake has been made.

Another possible explanation for the increased number of diagnoses is that societal expectations regarding behavior have changed, and persons with ADHD are likely to come into conflict with those expectations, resulting in them seeking diagnosis and treatment. For instance, a child with ADHD might have fewer problems getting along in an elementary school classroom that allowed children to move about freely and that emphasized a variety of social and developmental activities along with more conventional academic learning. The same child, placed in a classroom that demanded students sit at their desks for long periods, working silently and independently, and that placed great emphasis on academic achievement as indicated by standardized tests, might find it impossible to cope with the demands placed on them, and might thus be identified as uncooperative and disruptive. In the first case, the child's parents would have no reason to seek an ADHD evaluation for them, while in the second case, they might.

3. Who is diagnosed with ADHD?

There is no special category of people who can "get" ADHD, although diagnoses of ADHD are more common in some groups of people than in others. In the United States, ADHD is most commonly diagnosed in childhood—in fact, it is one of the most common childhood disorders in the United States—and can persist into adolescence and adulthood. In fact, according to the National Institute of Mental Health, in about one-third of individuals diagnosed with ADHD in childhood also have ADHD as adults.

According to data from the National Survey of Children's Health (NSCH), a survey designed to gather data about the physical and emotional health of children from birth through age 17 sponsored by the Maternal and Child Health Bureau of the Health Resources and Services Administration (HRSA), for children with a current diagnosis of ADHD, the median age of onset was 6 years. This means that half the children with ADHD had an age of onset (beginning of ADHD symptoms, not necessarily age at diagnosis) below 6 years, and half above 6 years. Age of diagnosis varied with the severity of the condition, suggesting that parents whose children had more severe symptoms took them for an evaluation earlier, resulting in diagnosis at a younger age. For children with severe ADHD, the median age of diagnosis was 4 years, while for children with moderate ADHD it was 6 years, and for those with mild ADHD, it was 7 years.

In each year for which we have data, more male than female children are diagnosed with ADHD in the United States. In 2003, for instance, 11.0 percent of boys aged 17 and under had been diagnosed with ADHD at some point in their lives, as compared to 4.4 percent of girls. The percentage of both boys and girls with an ADHD diagnosis has increased over the years, but the pattern of males being substantially more likely to have an ADHD diagnosis remains consistent. In 2007, 13.2 percent of boys and 5.6 percent of girls had received an ADHD diagnosis, while in 2011, 15.1 percent of boys and 6.7 percent of girls had received an ADHD diagnosis.

We don't know exactly why this persistently observed pattern of more males than females being diagnosed with ADHD exists. One possibility is that the data is simply revealing the straightforward reality that ADHD is simply more common among males than females. Many conditions and disorders occur more commonly in one gender than the other, so this would not be a surprising result. More complicated possibilities include that many people still believe that ADHD only occurs in boys, and thus if the same symptoms were displayed by a boy and a girl, the boy but not the girl would be referred for evaluation. Another possibility is that the symptoms of ADHD describe typical behaviors more commonly shown by boys, while the condition may produce different symptoms in girls that have not been incorporated into the diagnostic criteria of ADHD. Again, this is not an uncommon occurrence in the official diagnostic criteria for medical and psychiatric conditions, which are often based primarily on symptoms typical of men. A third possibility is that ADHD in boys is most often characterized by behaviors that are disruptive to a classroom setting or to home life and thus demand attention resulting in a referral to a specialist and ultimately a diagnosis, while in girls the condition results in quieter behaviors which are more easily overlooked and thus do not result in a referral and a diagnosis.

The proportion of children with ADHD diagnoses varies by race and ethnic group, although, as with gender differences in diagnosis, this could be due to many factors. Potential explanations include unequal access to counseling and medical services, differential judgments about the same behavior by authority figures (for instance, a teacher punishing a Black child that misbehaves more severely than a white child exhibiting the same behavior), the presence of comorbidities (diseases or other conditions that the child also has) that vary by race and ethnic groups, and differing beliefs in different cultural groups regarding ADHD. According to the Centers for Disease Control and Prevention (CDC), recent surveys found that ADHD diagnoses were most common among Black children (12 percent), with slightly lower rate of diagnosis among white children (8 percent) and an even lower rate of diagnosis among Asian children (3 percent).

ADHD diagnosis rates also vary by state, according to the CDC, with the lowest rate in Nevada (5.1 percent), followed by Colorado (6.3 percent) and California (6.7 percent). The highest rates of ADHD diagnosis were found in Louisiana (16.6 percent) and Mississippi (15.8 percent). There are many possible reasons for these differences found in diagnosis, as there are for the differences found in diagnosis rates nationally, but there is no definitive explanation for them at this time. Possible reasons for the differences observed include the different population makeup (by race, income level, etc.) found in each state, differences in expectations for how children should behave, and different access to resources that would potentially lead to an ADHD diagnosis or to other means of dealing with observed behaviors.

Separate surveys of adolescents and adults have also found different proportions of the US population with an ADHD diagnosis. There are many possible reasons for these observed differences, beginning with the fact that each survey is conducted with a sample of individuals, and the rate of diagnosis can be expected to differ somewhat among different samples. A more important reason is what is called the "cohort effect" in population statistics. A cohort is a group of people born at about the same time—for instance, everyone born in 1980, or everyone born in the years between 1975 and 1985. Because ADHD diagnoses have become more common over the years, and the recognition that older children and adults can have ADHD is relatively recent, it's not surprising that people born in an earlier generation might have a lower rate of diagnosis for ADHD, regardless of what symptoms they may have experienced, than people born more recently, in an era when ADHD diagnoses have become more common.

Given those caveats, according to the National Institute for Mental Health, lifetime prevalence of ADHD (meaning that the person got an ADHD diagnosis at any point in their life) was 8.7 percent for American adolescents aged 13 through 18 years. As with children, diagnosed ADHD is more common among male adolescents (13.0 percent) than among female adolescents (4.2 percent). Diagnostic rates also differ by racial and ethnic groups among adolescents: 9.3 percent of Black adolescents have an ADHD diagnosis, as compared to 8.9 percent of white adolescents, 8.5 percent of Hispanic adolescents, and 5.6 percent of those in other racial/ethnic categories (including Asian). Looking at adults aged 18–44, the CDC states that 4.4 percent report having a current ADHD (meaning having current symptoms associated with ADHD), with 8.1 percent having received an ADHD diagnosis at some point in their life. As with children and adolescents, males (5.4 percent) were more likely than females (3.2 percent) to have current ADHD. Unlike the younger age groups, however, current ADHD was most common among non-Hispanic whites (5.4 percent), as compared to 3.6 percent for "other" racial ethnic categories (including Asians), 2.1 percent for Hispanics, and 1.9 percent for Blacks.

It's more difficult to determine rates of ADHD internationally, due to differences in national cultures, availability of medical and psychiatric care, and differences in how data is collected and reported. However, some studies have estimated that about 7.2 percent of children globally have had ADHD at some point in their lives, with a higher prevalence in North America and the Middle East, and a lower prevalence in Africa and Asia. The finding that ADHD is more common in boys than girls is also seen in studies outside the United States, and most studies looking at ADHD incidence over time have seen an increase in diagnoses over the years.

4. What are some risk factors for ADHD?

While the ultimate causes of ADHD remain uncertain, several risk factors for ADHD have been identified. In medical terms, a risk factor means something that increases the chance of developing a particular disease or condition. Sometimes the connection between risk factors and a disease or condition is straightforward and well established, with strong biological explanations for the relationship, as the link between cigarette smoking and lung cancer. However, sometimes a risk factor is identified through statistical studies without a clear understanding of why the factor should increase the risk, and without sufficient evidence to establish a causal relationship. Because ADHD is less well understood than many conditions, most risk factors for ADHD fall into the latter category—a relationship between the factor and the occurrence of ADHD has been observed, but the exact reasons for that relationship are not well-understood. The fact that something has been identified as a risk factor for ADHD does not necessarily mean that the factor causes ADHD or that it has to be present in order for ADHD to occur—it may simply mean that a statistical relationship has been observed between the presence of the risk factor and ADHD.

Premature birth has been identified as a risk factor for ADHD, since premature babies are likely to have low or very low birth weights, and low or very low birth weight is associated with 2.4 to 4 times the occurrence of ADHD as compared to children of normal birth weight. Maternal malnutrition is associated with increased ADHD in children, as is fetal exposure to alcohol and maternal exposure to some pesticides. Children from mothers who had type 1 or type 2 diabetes during the pregnancy are more likely than average to be diagnosed with ADHD, and one study found that mothers with asthma are more likely than average to have children with ADHD. Exposure to heavy metals, including mercury and lead, has also been identified as a risk factor for ADHD, and some studies have found links between ADHD and elevated blood levels of various other heavy metals, including cadmium, manganese, cobalt, nickel, copper, molybdenum, tin, and barium. Low levels of one or more specific heavy metals, including manganese, chromium, and zinc, have also been found to be more common in children with ADHD than in the general population.

A number of environmental factors have also been associated with ADHD. Stressful maternal events during pregnancy, such as the death of a close relative, have been linked to increased likelihood of ADHD in boys. Exposure to neglect or sexual abuse in childhood has been found to be related to increased risk for ADHD even after accounting for factors such as race, ethnicity, and income. Family poverty and related factors such as parental unemployment and low levels of parental education are associated with increased risk of ADHD in children. Factors such as parental substance abuse, parental criminality, and residential instability have also been liked to increased risk of ADHD in children. In contrast, strong levels of family cohesion and community support have been associated with lower rates of ADHD in children.

5. Do the brains of people with ADHD differ from the brains of people without the condition?

Numerous studies have found differences between the brains of people with and without ADHD, both as measured indirectly by an individual's performance on psychological tests, and as measured directly by examination of brain structure and function using medical imaging techniques. Many studies have found differences in intellectual functioning between persons with and without ADHD, but such differences tend to be small and thus not useful for diagnosis. In addition, these differences may change over time, and may be due not to the ADHD directly but due to environmental factors (for instance, lower intellectual functioning as a result of being placed in special education for reasons of misbehavior), or due to reasons related to the way these qualities are measured (e.g., not being able to maintain concentration over the testing period) rather than the quality supposedly being measured (e.g., intelligence).

Some studies have found that people with ADHD score lower on IQ tests and on tests of typical school subjects like reading, spelling, and arithmetic, but such differences tend to be small and often not clinically significant. Some studies have found that people with ADHD do less well on measures of abstract problem solving, working memory, and verbal memory, while others have found small associations with ADHD and a preference for immediate rewards and a tendency to make risky decisions. Notably, many studies found that these impairments decreased with age, suggesting that people with ADHD find ways to cope with or work around these tendencies as they mature. Also, several studies have demonstrated that some ADHD deficits, such as those in working memory and impulse control, can be addressed through cognitive training.

MRI (magnetic resonance imaging, a method to create images of soft tissue such as the brain, and to study brain functioning) studies have found some physical differences in the brains of people with and without ADHD. For instance, children with ADHD have been found to have, on average, reduced cortical surface and reduced cortical thickness in some regions of the brain. Studies have also found that in children with ADHD, some areas of the brain were smaller than in the brains of children without ADHD. However, the differences observed in these studies were small and subtle, and were present only in children, not in adolescents or adults.

Other MRI studies have found differences in the activation of brain areas in those with and without ADHD. One finding replicated multiple times is that people with ADHD show less activation in regions responsible for inhibitory control, including the right inferior frontal cortex, supplementary motor area, and basal ganglia. Diffusion tensor imaging, a technique related to MRI, has found that ADHD and non-ADHD subjects commonly differ in activation of the corpus callosum, right sagittal stratum, and left tapetum, suggesting difficulties in connecting the activity of the two brain hemispheres and in areas involved with attention and control.

Some studies have also used imaging techniques to compare persons with ADHD to those with other psychiatric diseases and conditions. Compared to people with OCD (obsessive-compulsive disorder), people with ADHD have reduced structural gray matter volume in their basal ganglia and insula and a smaller hippocampus volume; the latter was shown to be related to IQ differences. ADHD patients were also differentiated from those having autism spectrum disorder (ASD), as the ASD patients tended to have reduced structural gray matter volume in the medial frontal area, while the ADHD patients did not.

Scientists have also studied differences in the electrical activity of the brain, as measured by quantitative electroencephalography (qEEG), a technique based on mathematical analysis of digital signals from an electroencephalogram (EEG). The most common measure used in the United States is the scalp vertex theta/beta ratio (TBR), a ratio of theta activity divided by beta activity as measured at the scalp vertex. The TBR is a noninvasive test that has been promoted as a means of diagnosing ADHD, but the American Academy of Neurology (AAN) cautions that the results of this test should not replace a standard clinical evaluation, and that studies of the TBR as a diagnostic tool have produced contradictory results. The AAN therefore does not recommend use of the TBR as a diagnostic tool, and many health insurance companies in the United States won't pay for it because they consider it to be experimental rather than a standard clinical tool.

6. Is there a genetic component to ADHD?

Many researchers believe there is a strong genetic component to ADHD, although the exact nature of that relationship is not entirely known. Family, twin, and adoption studies are one source of information in this regard, as they are a common way for researchers to separate out the influence of genetic factors in a disease or condition from environmental influences. Having a sibling with ADHD increases the probability that an individual will have ADHD, and the relationship is stronger with biological siblings than with an adopted child raised in the same household. Twin studies have found heritability indexes for ADHD ranging from about 50 percent to almost 100 percent, with an average of 70–80 percent, meaning that co-occurrence of ADHD in monozygotic (identical) twin pairs is much more common than in dizygotic twin pairs, suggesting a strong role for genetic makeup in ADHD.

Numerous studies have looked at relationships between a person's genetic makeup and the likelihood they will have ADHD. Many of these studies are genomic, meaning the researchers have looked at the genome (the entire set of genes in a person's body) of large numbers of people to find differences between those with and without ADHD. It is generally agreed today that ADHD is polygenic, meaning it is associated with numerous variants in individual genes, each variant adding a small increase of risk for ADHD, with no single genetic variant solely responsible for the condition. Many of the genes being studied in relation to ADHD have also been implicated in increased risk for psychiatric conditions such as schizophrenia, bipolar disorder, autism spectrum disorder, and eating and substance use disorders.

The genes associated with increased risk of ADHD tend to be those involved in processes such as transmitting impulses between neurons (neurotransmission) and the creation of synapses (synaptogenesis) which allow neurons to exchange chemical and electrical signals. The gene responsible for creating BDNF (brain-derived neurotrophic factor, which plays an important role in neuronal development) is an example of one such gene. Some studies have found associations with low levels of BDNF and ADHD, and pharmacological treatments are available to regulate BDNF levels. Other studies have found a relationship between BDNF levels and ADHD in males only, and some studies have found no relationship at all, although this latter result could have been influenced by factors specific to the studies in question, such as the time of day in which the samples were collected (BDNF levels fluctuate through the day).

Another gene widely studied in relation to ADHD is that which contains instructions for making the dopamine transporter DAT. Dopamine is a neurotransmitter that carries signals between neurons and plays important roles in thought and behavior. DAT is responsible for dopamine reuptake, and studies have found that persons with ADHD tend to have lower levels of DAT than people without ADHD. Two common pharmacological treatments for ADHD, amphetamines and methylphenidate, both target the functioning of the dopamine system.

7. Is there a link between vaccines and ADHD?

There is no link between vaccines and ADHD, although some people believe there is. This belief very likely has its roots in an earlier belief, now thoroughly discredited, that childhood vaccines can cause autism. Medical science is clear on both points: there is no causal link between vaccines and ADHD, and no link between childhood vaccines and autism. Vaccines are an important tool in the arsenal of modern medicine, and failing to get the recommended vaccinations on schedule exposes not only the unvaccinated individual but also those around them to the risk of diseases and complications that could have been prevented by the vaccine.

It's common for people in the United States to receive many vaccines over the course of their life. Children generally receive a series of vaccinations protecting them against deadly diseases like polio, diphtheria, and tetanus, as well as against what used to be called "diseases of childhood" like measles, mumps, and rubella (German measles), which can have serious side effects like brain damage and hearing loss. Older adults commonly get vaccines to protect them against diseases like pneumonia and shingles, and many people get an annual flu shot to protect them against seasonal influenza. During the Covid-19 pandemic, researchers produced effective vaccines against this disease in record time, and millions of people around protected themselves by getting vaccinated.

The fact that many Americans have never experienced potentially deadly or crippling diseases like polio or diphtheria, or even met someone who has had them, is a tribute to the life-saving benefits of vaccines. Most people understand the benefits of vaccination and get the standard vaccinations on the schedule recommended by their physician. However, some people have found the number of recommended vaccinations alarming (granted, the number has increased since some of today's adults were children), noted the rise in diagnoses of autism among children, and thought there might be a causal link. The MMR (measles, mumps, rubella) vaccine became a particular target of suspicion, with some claiming that the vaccine caused autism, but this is an example of correlation (an observed relationship between two things) not being causal. In fact, this belief may have its origins in the fact that the age at which the MMR vaccine is administered (12–18 months) is often the time when disorders like autism first become noticeable, so the coincidence of timing rather than any causal relationship between vaccines and autism explains why might seem to be related.

The vaccines-autism link was promoted by the former British physician Andrew Wakefield, who published research in a prestigious medical journal, *The Lancet*, purporting to establish a link between autism and the MMR vaccine. This "research" was later withdrawn under suspicions of fraud, research misconduct, and conflicts of interest, and Wakefield forfeited his medical license. Numerous large-scale studies have found no link between autism and vaccines, and the supposed causal agent, thimerosal (a preservative compound which contains mercury), not only has been demonstrated to be safe in the dosages used. It is also worth noting that thimerosal contains ethyl mercury, which is quickly eliminated from the body, unlike methyl mercury, which is sometimes found in seafood and can accumulate in the body.

Concerns about a connection between the thimerosal in vaccines and ADHD have also been raised, and the question is not illegitimate because exposure to heavy metals such as mercury is a risk factor for ADHD. However, thimerosal has not been used in vaccines administered in the United States since 2001, and it has been demonstrated to be safe in the amounts contained in vaccines. Given the amount of publicity granted over the years to false beliefs about vaccines causing autism or ADHD, it may not be surprising that some people still believe there is a connection. However, the verdict is clear on this issue: vaccines do not cause autism, they do not cause ADHD, and concerns about either condition should not prevent anyone from getting the recommended vaccinations on the schedule recommended by medical experts. One unfortunate consequence of people refusing to have their children vaccinated has been sporadic outbreaks of vaccine-preventable diseases like measles and diphtheria, which can have serious consequences to a child's health.

8. What are some diseases and conditions that commonly co-occur with ADHD?

It is common for people with ADHD to also experience additional diseases or conditions, which are known in medicine as comorbidities or coexisting conditions. These comorbidities can be either psychiatric, like autism or learning disorders, or nonpsychiatric, like diabetes or asthma. There is no implication of causality when discussing comorbidities—the term simply means that an individual has more than one disease or condition at the same time. For individuals suffering one or more comorbidities, it is important that they receive appropriate treatment for each disease or condition as well as for ADHD.

Psychiatric comorbidities are very common among people with ADHD, although overlap in symptoms and the specific requirements to identify each disease may make it difficult for an individual to receive a correct diagnosis. For instance, *DSM-IV* (the *Diagnostic and Statistical Manual of Mental Disorders*, which is the standard authority in the United States for psychiatric diagnoses) did not allow dual diagnosis of ADHD and autism spectrum disorder (ASD), so anyone diagnosed with ADHD when this manual was in use (1994–2013) by definition could not also be diagnosed with ASD. The newest edition, *DSM-5*, does allow for dual diagnosis of ADHD and ASD, so anyone evaluated under the old system might want to schedule a re-evaluation if they believe they may have ASD. One national study found that 59 percent of children diagnosed with ASD also had either a diagnosis of ADHD as well or diagnoses of both ADHD and a learning difficulty. This demonstrates that not only can these conditions occur together but it's not uncommon for them to do so. It also demonstrates that it is possible for clinicians to differentiate among these different disorders.

People with ADHD are often diagnosed with learning disorders as well, with some studies finding the rate of comorbidity to be over 90 percent, while others have found rates as low as 10 percent. The most common learning disabilities to co-occur with ADHD are those related to writing (such as dysgraphia), although disabilities relating to reading, math, and spelling have also been identified. Persons with ADHD also have a higher than average rate of tic disorders such as Tourette's syndrome, which is characterized by involuntary movements (tics) and vocalizations. Looking from the opposite direction, one study found that 55 percent of individuals diagnosed with Tourette's syndrome also had ADHD.

Depression is more common in young people with ADHD than in those without it, with rates of 12 percent to 50 percent for co-occurrence found in different studies. Depressive symptoms often occur several years after the onset of ADHD and may be related to negative experiences in dealing with ADHD as well as to independent causes. Pediatric bipolar disorder has been linked to ADHD in many studies, although the mechanisms of comorbidity are not well understood. Anxiety disorders are common in persons with ADHD, with co-occurrence rates estimated from 15 percent to 35 percent in various studies. As with depression, anxiety disorders may both have independent origins from ADHD and be worsened by the stress of living with ADHD.

Externalizing disorders like oppositional defiant disorder (ODD) and conduct disorder (CD) commonly co-occur with ADHD, with some studies finding that 30 percent to 50 percent of persons with ADHD also have ODD or CD, with these comorbidities more common in boys than girls. Individuals diagnosed with both ADHD and CD are at increased risk for adult antisocial personality disorder, are more likely to engage in criminal behaviors and drug abuse, and are more likely to drop out of or be expelled from school than individuals with ADHD alone.

Persons with ADHD are more likely than the general population to be affected by certain nonpsychiatric diseases and conditions. Several studies have found that adolescents and adults with ADHD suffer from type 2 diabetes at a rate much higher than the general population, and other studies have found that persons who have both ADHD and type 1 diabetes tend to have poorer metabolic control than type 1 diabetes patients without ADHD, and to be at increased risk for complications such as diabetic ketoacidosis. Whether these last two findings are the result of people with ADHD having a more difficult time organizing their diet and care schedule (a problem which could be improved through education) or if there are additional biological factors at play, is not certain. Although not everyone considers obesity a problem or concern, it is a risk factor for type 2 diabetes and some other conditions, so it is worth noting that persons with untreated ADHD are more likely to be obese than the general population, while this effect is not seen in persons receiving appropriate ADHD treatment.

Associations have been found between allergies and related diseases, including asthma and eczema with ADHD. However, research in this field has generally been done by looking at people with asthma and/or eczema and then determining how many have ADHD, with the consistent finding that people with allergy-related diseases are more likely than the general public to have ADHD. Both men and women with ADHD are at increased risk of being diagnosed with psoriasis, with the risk greater for women than men. Some studies have found increased sleep disorders among people with ADHD, and some have not, but surveys of people with ADHD have found that they report difficulties with sleep at a higher rate than does the general population.

9. Why do some people think ADHD isn't a real condition?

Medical and psychology professionals today are generally in agreement that ADHD is a real condition, with specific diagnostic criteria and effective treatments available. ADHD is included in the fifth edition of the *Diagnostic and Statistical Manual* (*DSM-5*) of the American Psychiatric Association, and conditions with symptoms similar to what we now term ADHD have been included in the *DSM* since the second edition was published in 1968. Many other countries and international organizations, including the European Union and the World Health Organization, also recognize ADHD as a condition with specific diagnostic criteria and available treatments. Despite this consensus, some individuals believe that ADHD is not "real," but is simply a medicalization of normal behavior, a cash grab by pharmaceutical companies and medical professionals, or an excuse for bad behavior.

One reason some people may doubt the existence of ADHD is because, as is the case with many psychiatric conditions, there is no simple blood or imaging test available to make a diagnosis of ADHD. Instead, the diagnostic process depends on the clinical judgment of a medical specialist and is based on observation, interviews, and psychological testing. In the absence of an objective physical test comparable to the presence of bacteria in the bloodstream, or a fracture on an X-ray, some people believe that it's easy to "fake" an ADHD evaluation to get a diagnosis. This belief has been bolstered by news reports of students being coached on how to get an ADHD diagnosis in order to receive more time on exams or the opportunity to take the SAT outside the usual testing schedule. There is also a belief among some people that some parents may engage in "doctor shopping" until they find one willing to give their child the desired diagnosis, and people who believe this may point to the increasing number of children diagnosed with ADHD, as well as the fact that ADHD diagnoses are more common among the affluent that in the general population, as evidence for this belief. In fact, we know that diagnoses of ADHD are increasing in part because people are more aware of it, and also because access to health care in the United States may be dependent on income, people with more money may well access more and better care, and hence be more likely to receive a diagnosis. Neither of those points provides any evidence that ADHD does not exist or that most diagnoses are fraudulent.

As is also the case with many psychiatric conditions, at least some of the symptoms of ADHD, such as inattentiveness and impulsiveness, have been experienced by many people. It's not uncommon, after all, to experience your attention drifting away when you are bored, or to occasionally fail to complete your work on time or exactly to specifications. The difference between these common experiences and ADHD is that the diagnostic criteria for ADHD requires professional evaluation and consideration of multiple factors, including the frequency and severity of the symptoms, whether they are interfering with the individual's normal daily functioning, and whether there are other explanations for the symptoms observed. Although there may have been cases in which a patient successfully got an ADHD diagnosis through deception or bribery, that doesn't mean that everyone diagnosed with ADHD is a faker, any more than the fact that one person telling a lie means that no one is ever truthful.

The increase in ADHD diagnoses, and the use of medicines prescribed to people with ADHD, is another reason that some people think ADHD is an invented condition. However, the increase in diagnoses can be explained by parents, teachers, and medical professionals becoming more aware of this condition, and the availability of drugs and other treatments that can improve the lives of ADHD patients. The fact that ADHD sometimes appears to be a "condition of privilege" (meaning diagnosis is more common among white, financially secure families) doesn't invalidate the diagnostic process—instead, it suggests that having the knowledge and resources to access appropriate care is not evenly distributed through the population (which is a fact, at least in the United States). And if some people abuse ADHD drugs (e.g., taking drugs prescribed to someone else in order to feel "sharper" before an exam), that doesn't invalidate the experience of people who were appropriately prescribed drugs for ADHD and use them as directed. In short, people who claim ADHD is not a real condition are making an inappropriate statement based on a lack of information and understanding, and such opinions should not prevent anyone from seeking expert help if they feel they or their child have ADHD, nor should it prevent them from following the treatment plan prescribed (to be adjusted as necessary in consultation with a medical professional).

2

Characteristics of ADHD

10. What are the most common symptoms of ADHD?

Different people with ADHD may have different sets of symptoms, but there are also certain commonalities that are characteristic of ADHD. Not every person with ADHD will have all the symptoms that are officially recognized, and not everyone who has some of the symptoms will necessarily be diagnosed with ADHD. Most of the symptoms associated with ADHD are based on observations of behavior rather than physical tests (there is no blood test which can detect ADHD, for instance), which is one reason professional expertise is required to make a diagnosis.

ADHD symptoms fall into three main categories: inattention, hyperactivity, and impulsivity. Inattention means it is difficult for a person to keep their focus on a task and to stay organized, when such problems are not due to lack of comprehension or deliberate choice. In other words, a person suffering from inattention may be trying their best to work hard on a task (such as completing math homework for school or writing a report for their job) which they are capable of doing, and yet they find themselves unable to stay focused on the task and to organize their efforts, resulting in a finished product far inferior to what they were capable of producing. Inattentive symptoms may easily be overlooked and the resulting poor performance attributed to lack of talent ("she's just not good at math") or lack of effort ("he'd rather play than focus on his work").

Symptoms of hyperactivity, as the name implies (in medicine, "hyper" is means "above normal"), include excessive movement, with "excessive" defined according to the expectations of a particular context. For instance, it is normal behavior to run on the playground during recess but running around the classroom while the teacher is delivering a lesson would not be appropriate, and thus the latter but not the former might be considered an indication of hyperactivity. Symptoms of hyperactivity can be less obvious as well, manifesting in behaviors such as fidgeting, tapping a pencil, or talking when it is not appropriate. Hyperactive behaviors tend to be visible and to disrupt the lives of both the hyperactive person and those around them, and are thus likely to draw attention and disapproval, particularly in a formal classroom setting. While it's good that hyperactive behaviors tend to be noticed, and thus are more likely to result in a referral, it's unfortunate that they be treated as signs of poor discipline and punished as misbehavior.

Symptoms of impulsivity including acting without thinking and failing to display appropriate levels of self-control, given age and developmental level. A person suffering from impulsivity may find it difficult to organize themselves and work consistently on a project or an assignment, may have trouble conversing because they tend to speak before waiting for the other speakers to finish, and may intrude on others' conversations or activities without realizing that they are doing so. Symptoms of impulsivity and hyperactivity may appear similar and often occur in the same person. In adults, symptoms of impulsivity may be less obvious, but can result in difficulties in making and carrying out long-term projects and a tendency to make important decisions without thinking through all the consequences.

Many people have exhibited one or more of these symptoms at some point in their life. However, the difference between any person making the occasional bad decision and a person who is diagnosed with ADHD has a lot to do with the severity and frequency of the symptoms and whether they interfere with the person's normal life. For people with ADHD, symptoms of inattention, hyperactivity, or impulsivity, or some combination of the three, occur more frequently, are more severe, and interfere with the person's normal functioning in age-appropriate activity such as attending school, socializing, or working.

11. Does ADHD present differently in males and females?

More males than females have been diagnosed with ADHD, and this pattern has been consistent for years. While it is possible that the occurrence of ADHD differs by gender, as is true for some medical conditions, it is also possible that boys displaying symptoms of ADHD are simply more likely to be referred for evaluation and to receive a diagnosis of ADHD than are girls displaying symptoms that would also qualify them for a diagnosis. Differences in referral and diagnosis rates could therefore be related to the type and severity of symptoms exhibited, with girls' symptoms more likely to be overlooked or mislabeled than those displayed by the boys.

Another factor to keep in mind is that much of the early work on identifying and diagnosing ADHD was based on observing boys, and that the symptoms chosen to define an ADHD diagnosis were based on the behavior exhibited by those boys. The possibility that ADHD might manifest itself differently in girls was not a focus of the earliest research on ADHD, which instead focused on describing the characteristics of the primarily male patients observed. This is a phenomenon often seen in medicine, with diagnostic criteria for conditions from HIV infection to heart attacks often based on symptoms commonly experienced by men, so that different symptoms commonly experienced by women may not be included in the diagnostic criteria for years, if at all.

Modern research indicates that ADHD symptoms often differ between males and females, with males more likely to display hyperactive and impulsive symptoms, and girls more likely to experience inattentive symptoms. This could be due to an overall tendency often observed between males and females (whether based on biology, socialization, or some combination of the two is an open question) that internalizing behavior (withdrawing from a social context, blaming oneself, trying to please others at the expense of one's own desires) is more commonly displayed by girls and women in the United States, while externalizing behavior (activity, disruption) is more commonly displayed by boys and men.

Given these facts, it's not hard to understand why boys and men, whose ADHD more often results in externalizing behaviors that can disrupt a classroom or workplace or social context, would be more likely to be identified as having a problem that needed to be dealt with, resulting in referral for evaluation and diagnosis. Girls and women, whose inattentive symptoms result hamper their ability to learn and to function in a social or workplace context, but which would not cause a disruption that would disturb others, could be easily overlooked, so that the individuals affected are never referred for evaluation and diagnosis. Girls with ADHD are more likely to report experiencing depression and anxiety than are boys or non-ADHD female controls, possibly due to a tendency among girls and women to engage in internalizing behaviors, but anxiety or depression is not currently included in the criteria for ADHD diagnosis.

12. Does ADHD present differently in children and adults?

ADHD was originally defined based on observation and study of children, primarily boys, and was originally believed to only occur in childhood. The belief in the early years of the awareness of this condition was that children who were diagnosed with ADHD in childhood would simply "grow out" of this condition as they matured. We know today that this is not true, although adults with ADHD may well have learned how to control the overt and disruptive manifestations of the condition. For instance, an adult who disrupted an office by running and yelling would not stay employed for long, so most people learn to suppress such tendencies, even if the impulses underlying them still remain. Adults with ADHD who did not receive a diagnosis in childhood may not realize they have this condition, but it may be interfering with their daily functioning and ability to achieve their full potential in ways they do not realize. Fortunately, awareness of ADHD in adults is increasing and many people have received a first-time diagnosis as adults, followed up by appropriate treatment.

Typical ADHD symptoms in adults include difficulties in organizing their work tasks, regularly forgetting appointments and deadlines, and finding it difficult to carry on ordinary tasks like getting to work on time or concentrating once they get there. Adults with ADHD may feel constantly restless or try to do too many things at once, and may have difficulty in carrying on conversations or engaging in social relationships because they find behaviors such as taking turns when speaking to be difficult. They may also have a history of making snap decisions in important matters (such as buying a new car or quitting a job), and to be constantly chasing after new opportunities rather than completing the responsibilities they have already taken on.

As with childhood behaviors typical of ADHD, adult symptoms are common to many people from time to time, so the important criteria include the frequency and severity of the symptoms and whether they interfere with an individual's functioning. Difficulties with executive function, which often occur in people with ADHD, are particularly problematic in adulthood because it is generally assumed that adults should be able to break down complex tasks into components, make plans to complete the necessary parts, and carry out those plans without a lot of external support. Inability to do so may make it impossible for someone to advance in their career and may result in frustration and anxiety because the person with ADHD may not realize why their performance consistently falls short of the expectations of themselves and others. Besides internalizing blame for something that is not truly their fault, adults with ADHD may be judged harshly by others, with their behaviors criticized as personal deficiencies ("he doesn't care enough to do a good job" or "she never sees a task through to its conclusion") rather than as symptoms of a condition that could be treated.

13. What are the executive functions, and how do they relate to ADHD?

Executive functions are cognitive skills that allow people to control and coordinate their other cognitive abilities and behaviors. Three main executive functions have been identified: working memory, cognitive flexibility, and inhibition control. Together, the executive functions perform tasks analogous to that of a person holding an executive job in a business context: the executive is tasked with making long-term plans and monitoring the company's progress toward them, while lower-level employees carry out the necessary tasks to fulfill those plans and respond to feedback from the executive. A deficiency in the executive functions may be termed executive dysfunction, and people with executive dysfunction tend to have difficulties with tasks such as planning, problem-solving, and task completion. In adulthood, and to some extent in the educational system, we expect individuals to act as the executives of their own lives, setting their own goals, making plans to reach them, monitoring their progress, and making corrections as necessary. As with other aspects of ADHD, difficulties with executive function may be mischaracterized as negative character traits or antisocial behaviors such as laziness, lack of caring, or lack of ambition, rather than as symptoms of a condition that requires appropriate treatment.

Working memory refers to the information held in the "front of your mind" which is easily accessible while you perform a specific cognitive task. For instance, you may hold a phone number in your working memory long enough to dial it. Working memory is distinguished from long-term memory, which refers to the vast body of knowledge and experiences you have stored in your mind over the course of your life and which you may need to recall to your working memory in order to complete a specific task. For instance, to solve a physics problem you may need to recall a formula into your working memory and then apply it to the information you have. Working memory is necessary to succeed in school—a student must be able to call to mind important facts or techniques necessary to solve problems or understand a text they are reading, to use those facts or techniques effectively, and to remember what they have already done or what has already been said—and is also required for normal functioning in ordinary life.

Problems with working memory may manifest in many different ways, including difficulty following directions, a need to constantly reread text, and difficulties in staying engaged in class or on the job. Even the most ordinary tasks, such as carrying on a conversation, can be impacted because a person experiencing difficulties in working memory may not remember what has already been said, something that occurs automatically for most people. Children who have problems with working memory may struggle in school, despite high intelligence, and may have strained social relationships with their peers, who don't understand the cause of their difficulties. Many adults with ADHD struggle with one or more aspects of executive functioning, which often manifests itself as poor work performance despite having the desire to succeed as well as the necessary abilities and preparation.

Cognitive flexibility refers to the ability to shift your mind from one topic to another, or to switch between approaches to a topic or situation when it is beneficial to do so. Fluid or flexible thinking is a deliberate process controlled by the thinker, as compared to the involuntary switching and inability to concentrate on a topic sometimes experienced by people with ADHD. Flexible thinking enhances creative work but is also necessary for problem-solving in fields not normally thought of as creative or artistic. Creative thinking in mathematics, for instance, allows a student to try different approaches to a problem until they find one that works. For a scientist, creative thinking allows the incorporation of knowledge, techniques, and approaches from different fields, or from different people working into the same field, to come up with a new theory or new formulation of a problem.

Inhibition control is the ability to manage and control one's thoughts, emotions, and behaviors. We all experience inappropriate thoughts from time to time, as well as emotions that might better be left unexpressed, and perhaps also feel urges to behave in ways that are not appropriate to our immediate context. Most children learn inhibition control as part of the process of maturing and learning to act in a socially appropriate manner, so that as adults they are able to behave appropriately in different contexts. For people with ADHD, however, this learning process can be much more difficult.

There are two aspects of impulse control: behavioral control and interference. Behavioral control means you can recognize the impulse to do something as inappropriate or socially undesirable in the immediate context, and thus you choose to not act on the impulse. For instance, if someone verbally insults you, it's natural to want to insult them back, or to respond with physical violence, but the more mature response is to reply in a reasoned manner or simply ignore the insult and move on. What is considered appropriate behavior in a particular context may well be defined partly by cultural mores and customs and may differ depending on factors such as the age, gender, or social position of a person. Understanding that context is part of behavioral control: you have to know what is considered appropriate in order to be able to recognize and suppress behaviors that would be inappropriate. Lack of behavioral control can have serious consequences, from being expelled from school to being arrested, but can also have more subtle manifestations, such as an inability to thrive in a classroom or workplace environment.

Interference control means that you can manage your thoughts and maintain focus on what is important for the task at hand while not being distracted by what is not relevant. Young children are often easily distracted, but develop interference control as they grow and mature, and adults are generally expected to have strong interference control. Exerting interference control is often difficult for people with ADHD, and it's not an ability that necessary improves with age for them, which may result in them being labeled as immature. Because problems with interference control often have no physical manifestation, they may be overlooked in both children and adults, and poor performance on school or work tasks is ascribed to character flaws such as laziness or not caring enough to do the work properly.

14. What is hyperfocus, and how does it relate to ADHD?

Hyperfocus refers to a state in which a person is so completely absorbed in a task that they are unaware, or nearly unaware, of anything else. It is sometimes described as being completely "tuned in" to whatever one is doing (another phrasing is to be "locked on" to a task), to the point of ignoring your surroundings and anything happening in them. It's not uncommon to experience hyperfocus— if you've ever been so absorbed in a book or a video game that you didn't notice other people coming into the room, or didn't hear someone calling your name, you have experienced hyperfocus.

There is no agreed-upon scientific definition of hyperfocus, but the general concept has been studied in multiple contexts, including among people with ADHD, who seem to experience hyperfocus more commonly than the general population. One of the paradoxes of ADHD is that a person who is easily distractible and has difficulty maintaining attention on one type of task may display hyperfocus on another type of task, becoming so absorbed in it that they continue working on it for hours. Tasks that are perceived as fun or interesting, and are non-routine, are most likely to be the object of hyperfocus, and entering a state of hyperfocus is a voluntary behavior rather one that can be enforced by someone else.

Some research has focused on the negative aspects of hyperfocus, such as the difficulty in switching from one task to another, and the neglect of other aspects of the environment. Hyperfocus can be a problem in a school context if a student is expected to focus on what the teacher wants them to be doing at a particular moment, rather than what they are interested in (which is a typical expectation in a classroom). It can also be a problem if a student is expected to shift focus from task to task along with the rest of the class. For instance, a student hyperfocused on a task may resist leaving it just because the teacher has decided it's time to move on to the next lesson. Hyperfocus can also be a problem in a context where the social aspects are important, working on a group project, since someone in a state of hyperfocus may not notice or care about what anyone else is doing or thinking. Hyperfocus can also cause problems at work—in some businesses, being perceived as a "team player" is more important than the ability to create brilliant solutions to novel problems. In addition, the dynamics of some workplaces may mean that employees are expected to work on whatever they are assigned, rather than what interests them most, and to accept changes in their work assignments without protest.

Hyperfocus also has positive aspects, because many types of work, particularly in scientific and mathematical fields, benefit from long periods of intense focus. Important discoveries often come not from people working 9 to 5 on a variety of tasks but from someone having an almost obsessive focus on a particular problem that has captured their attention. Hyperfocus has been called a "superpower" because people who experience it generally get better and more efficient at whatever they are focused on, and if that focus is something useful or significant, society may well benefit as well. Some workplaces are recognizing the benefits of allowing periods of uninterrupted focus by establishing blocks of time within the work week during which no meetings are scheduled and no one is expected to respond to emails or phone calls. These innovations are relatively rare, however, and often apply only to certain workers (typically those involved in research at a high level), so the average employee is still expected to be willing and able to shift their attention on demand.

15. What is subthreshold ADHD?

A person with subthreshold ADHD has some of the symptoms of ADHD, but not enough to receive a diagnosis. It's important to understand that since there is no definitive physical test to diagnose ADHD, the clinical requirements for a diagnosis are not as absolute as they might be in, for instance, the diagnosis of an infectious disease through a blood test. Therefore, the lack of a formal ADHD diagnosis doesn't mean a person has no ADHD-related impairment. Someone with subthreshold ADHD may experience difficulties in their life related to ADHD and is deserving of appropriate treatment and accommodations to enable them to live their best life with as little impairment as possible. School systems that treat ADHD as a dichotomy—either a student has an official diagnosis of ADHD and is therefore entitled to accommodations or they don't have the diagnosis and should be treated just like everyone else—are doing a disservice to their students and taking the concept of ADHD diagnosis too literally.

Community studies of children have found that subthreshold ADHD occurs equally in boys and girls and is found more often in children from low-income families. Studies comparing children with an ADHD diagnosis, children with subthreshold ADHD, and healthy children without ADHD characteristics have found that children with subthreshold ADHD experience more serious functional impairments, as compared to children with no ADHD characteristics, although they experience fewer impairments than children with an ADHD diagnosis. Studies have also found that subthreshold ADHD symptoms in childhood are associated with poorer outcomes in adolescence, including lower academic achievement, poorer relationships with adults and peers, and lower self-esteem. These findings suggest it may be more useful to consider ADHD as existing on a spectrum, with some experiencing more and some experiencing less impairment, rather than as a dichotomy in which some have the condition and others do not, with no further nuance recognized within those two groups.

16. Are there links between diet and ADHD?

Many people have hypothesized that diet plays a role in ADHD. One particularly common belief is that consuming certain foods may hasten the appearance of ADHD symptoms or make those symptoms worse. Pediatric allergist Benjamin Feingold, a pioneer in this field, hypothesized that some artificial food additives and foods rich in salicylates might play a role in childhood hyperactivity. Other studies have looked at the effectiveness of limiting the foods consumed by ADHD patients (the "few foods diet," or FFD), eliminating foods with artificial food colorings (AFC) or other food additives from the diet, and supplementing the diet of ADHD patients with vitamins, minerals, and poly-unsaturated fatty acids (PUFA).

This line of research is fairly new, and there is no clear scientific consensus on the relationship between diet and ADHD. A review of the evidence from fourteen meta-analyses (analyses that combine the results from multiple studies) of dietary intervention in children with ADHD by Lidy M. Pelsser, Klaas Frankena, Jan Toorman, and Rob Rodrigues Pereir concludes that there is currently no evidence to support PUFA supplementation as an ADHD intervention, and more study was required to determine if AFC elimination could be useful in treating ADHD. However, they found substantial evidence supporting FFD as a treatment, particularly for children who do not respond to other types of treatment or who are too young to take ADHD medications. They recommend further research to better understand how an FFD interacts with ADHD in children and which subgroups respond best to this intervention.

Less research has been conducted on the relationship between diet and ADHD in adults, perhaps because until recently ADHD was considered primarily a condition of childhood. Some studies have found a relationship, others have not, and the evidence base is too small to conduct a meta-analysis such as that cited above by Pelsser and colleagues. The largest single study to date, conducted by Lin Li and colleagues, was based on almost 18,000 adults in Sweden. This study has the additional advantage of being conducted with twin pairs, allowing the researchers to estimate the heritability of certain traits (monozygotic twins are genetically identical, while dizygotic twins share about 50 percent of their genetic variation) and to separate genetic and environmental influences.

Li and colleagues found small positive correlations between ADHD and consumption of an unhealthy diet, and between ADHD and consumption of high levels of seafood, fat, sugar, and protein (meaning that people with higher levels of ADHD symptoms were more likely to consume more of these foods). They also found a small negative correlation between consumption of a healthy diet high in fruits and vegetables with ADHD symptoms (meaning those who ate healthy diets were less likely to have ADHD symptoms). Associations were stronger for inattention than for hyperactivity and impulsivity, although this could be related to the fact that adults with ADHD in general are less likely to display impulsivity and hyperactivity and more likely to display inattention. They also found high levels of heritability for inattention symptoms and a high sugar diet, inattention and an unhealthy diet, and hyperactivity and an unhealthy diet. While this is only one study and it was observational, so it cannot establish causality (it can't determine if food choices cause ADHD symptoms, if the symptoms cause the food choices, or if their co-occurrence is coincidental), it suggests that further research into the relationship between diet and ADHD in adults might produce useful results.

17. Can ADHD symptoms be affected by factors like stress or lack of sleep?

Many people have noticed that their ADHD symptoms (or those of their child) tend to appear and/or worsen under stressful conditions. "Stress" in this case means anything that requires a person to respond with attention or action. Stress is a normal part of life that can even be beneficial—for instance, many athletes perform their best in stressful conditions (such as in a championship game, as opposed to a practice session), and a small amount of stress can sharpen one's attention and lead to better performance at school or at work. However, too much stress can trigger a "fight-or-flight" response, which may have helped our ancestors survive but which may be inappropriate when taking an exam or speaking in public. This means that the amount and severity of stress is important, and too much stress can negatively affect anyone, including people with ADHD. This relationship is not just anecdotal: scientific research has found support for the suggestion that being under excessive stress is harmful for people with ADHD and can lead to the expression or worsening of ADHD symptoms.

Multiple studies have found an association between the experience of stress and adversity in early childhood and ADHD, measured both by the probability of an ADHD diagnosis and by the severity of symptoms. While the mechanism causing this relationship is unknown, some believe it is due to changes in the brain due to the experience of stressful events while the brain is most responsive to the environment. Some researchers have found that stressful events occurring before age 5 have greater impact in terms of ADHD than those occurring later in childhood and that the number of stressful events is important as well as their severity. Examples of childhood stress associated with ADHD diagnosis and severity include the experience of physical and sexual abuse, the experience of parental neglect, and exposure to parental domestic violence.

Research has also found that experiencing stress can worsen ADHD symptoms. For instance, a child who can normally manage their ADHD in a classroom setting may be triggered by the pressure of an important exam and display symptoms of hyperactivity and/or inattention, the former disrupting the classroom and the latter resulting in them doing poorly on the exam. Some scientists hypothesize that stress worsens ADHD symptoms because it affects the prefrontal cortex, the same part of the brain affected by ADHD, and which is responsible for executive control functions such as planning and managing attention and moderating behavior. Research also supports the suggestion that at least some adults with ADHD experience worsening of their symptoms in stressful situations, with the most common symptoms being inattention and slow mental processing (e.g., it might take longer than usual to perform calculations that are usually routine).

Although no one can expect to lead a life completely without stress, there are ways to control reactions to stress so they don't interfere with normal functioning. Any health professional providing care for a person with ADHD should be consulted for their advice regarding stress, but there are also many simple strategies that may help. One is to become aware of situations that are experienced as stressful by the person with ADHD, and to avoid those situations is possible. For instance, some people find loud noise to be stressful, while others experience stress when in a crowd of people, so they should avoid being in a noisy or crowded situation, perhaps by making specific changes to their daily routine. Students with an ADHD diagnosis can consult with the disability coordinator or guidance counselor at their school to discuss what accommodations might help them, such as being allowed to take exams in a quiet room with minimal distractions.

General advice on coping with stress may also be useful to people with ADHD. Many people find that eating a healthy diet, getting regular exercise, as well as getting sufficient sleep helps reduce their overall stress levels. Limiting time spent on social media can also be helpful, while spending more face-to-face time with people outside of a workplace or school context (e.g., by joining a club or sports team) may also help relieve stress. Choosing to give yourself a break, both in terms of not overscheduling yourself and in terms of being kind to yourself when you don't perform as well as you hoped, is also useful to reduce stress. Other target strategies when confronted with a stressful situation, such as controlling your breathing and engaging in positive self-talk, may also be useful, and a counselor or psychologist can help you learn these strategies and when to apply them.

Insufficient sleep, and poor quality sleep, can be stressful for anyone. Unfortunately, people with ADHD suffer from sleep disturbances at a higher rate than the general population, creating stress which may result in a worsening of their symptoms. Among the most common sleep problems are insomnia, difficulty in falling asleep, and waking multiple times per night. These patterns can prevent the sleeper from getting the rest they need, so they feel sleepy rather than refreshed upon awakening. Poor sleep may also lead to additional stress if a person starts to dread going to bed each night. Insufficient restful sleep is associated with a number of negative outcomes, including irritability, inattention, and fatigue, and can be dangerous if a person is so tired that they fall asleep spontaneously in a hazardous situation like driving a car. Sleep problems should be discussed with a health professional, but simple changes in routine (like observing a set bedtime and avoiding social media after a certain hour) can also be helpful.

18. What are the risks of ignoring ADHD symptoms?

Some people may feel that it is better to ignore the symptoms of ADHD than to seek diagnosis and treatment. This impulse is easy to understand, given that ADHD symptoms can vary widely in severity and may be similar to experiences and feelings shared with people who don't have ADHD. In addition, obtaining medical and psychological care costs money, and accessing care may require going through a series of bureaucratic requirements that seem daunting. Other motivations for avoiding getting ADHD symptoms evaluated include reluctance to have a label applied to oneself or one's child, mistrust of the medical and/or psychiatric professions, desire to avoid taking medications, and wishful thinking that the symptoms will end on their own if ignored.

Unfortunately, there are risks associated with not seeking expert advice when dealing with ADHD, and a lay person without medical or psychiatric training is not equipped to judge if particular symptoms or behaviors are caused by ADHD or not. ADHD symptoms do not necessarily go away on their own and the failure to manage ADHD can have lifetime consequences. Children with untreated ADHD may struggle in school, and the lack of a sound educational foundation will likely limit their choices of what type of work they are able to do as an adult. ADHD can also interfere with a child's ability to form healthy relationships with their peers and may result in them being isolated and bullied while not learning social skills that most children naturally pick up during their school years.

The consequences of failing to diagnose and treat ADHD symptoms can last into adulthood. Besides the education and social deficits that may be incurred in childhood and carry over into adult life, adults with ADHD are more likely to abuse tobacco, alcohol, and other drugs. Sometimes these behaviors are an attempt by an individual to self-medicate to cope with the problems caused by ADHD, in the absence of any truly effective help. Difficulty in functioning socially may cause a person to become bitter and isolated, or to accept abuse in a relationship because they have trouble relating to other people and are willing to accept a bad relationship rather than remain alone. Women with untreated ADHD are more likely to experience an unwanted pregnancy than those without ADHD, and sexually transmitted diseases are more common in people with untreated ADHD than in those without ADHD. Untreated ADHD can also lead to dangerous, thrill-seeking behavior, and the ability to safely drive a car, which is close to being a necessity in order to live a normal adult life in many parts of the United States, can be impaired by inattention and hyperactivity.

Independent of such tangible dangers of failing to seek diagnosis and treatment of ADHD, people with untreated ADHD may learn to not trust themselves because they become used to being disappointed with their own behavior. They may judge themselves harshly ("I'm so stupid," "I always do the wrong thing," etc.) because they don't understand how their brain works and how it influences their behavior. They may also accept a diminished version of their potential because they have failed so often in the past, without understanding why. While the process of ADHD diagnosis and treatment is not perfect, and it may take multiple efforts to find the right combination of therapies for any individual, the consequences of ignoring ADHD symptoms can be much more serious. In addition, undergoing evaluation with a trained health provider may uncover other conditions or impairments that can also be treated, and offers the opportunity for a person to understand themselves and their own mind better.

19. Are there other conditions that have similar characteristics to ADHD?

Some of the most common signs and symptoms associated with ADHD can occur for many reasons, and people without ADHD may experience many of them, complicating the evaluation process. The diagnosis of ADHD requires determining the severity and frequency of the symptoms—while anyone may experience inattention or restlessness from time to time, for instance, in people with ADHD these symptoms tend to be more frequent and more severe, and tend to cause problems for the individual, such as interfering with their ability to succeed in school or at their job. Evaluating an individual for ADHD also requires determining if some other condition or combination of factors could be the cause of the symptoms experienced. For instance, symptoms similar to ADHD may be caused by anxiety, depression, stress, or sleep disorders, so the diagnostic process will include evaluating whether those or similar conditions may in fact be responsible for the symptoms experienced.

Life circumstances are also important—for instance, if a person is experiencing a period of disturbed sleep due to problems at home, in school, or at work, that could result in symptoms similar to ADHD, even if the sleeping problems are not sufficiently severe to result in a clinical diagnosis of sleep disorder. Similarly, it's completely common for people to undergo periods of stress in their lives, and while the stress may not be at a level where clinical intervention is required, it can trigger behaviors similar to those seen in people with ADHD. It's important to remember that not only adults experience stress—although they may not know the word, children can be stressed by many factors, including parental discord, changing economic circumstances, pressure to do well in school, failure to fit in with peers or other family members, and bullying. These and similar circumstances may produce ADHD-like symptoms, but if a person has ADHD, their symptoms will persist even in times of low or nonexistent stress. Evaluation for potential learning disorders is also important, particularly for school-age children, since they may impede a student's performance in the classroom, leading to inattention, acting out, or other responses to frustration. Even if there are other factors at work, however, their effect may be magnified in a person who has ADHD, so the possibility of multiple causes for the same effect should always be considered.

It's important to get an ADHD evaluation from a trained professional because some of the symptoms of ADHD overlap with other clinical disorders. For instance, someone with bipolar disorder may have manic episodes characterized by symptoms similar to those of ADHD, such as hyperactivity and other inappropriate behavior. People on the autism spectrum may also display symptoms associated with ADHD, such as detachment from social situations or inappropriate social behaviors, including hyperactivity. Persons with sensory processing disorder, which is characterized by nonstandard (higher or lower than what is considered usual or normal) reactions to sensory input such as smell, taste, touch, or sound, may display symptoms similar to ADHD if they are exposed to something that disturbs them.

Physical limitations such as hearing or vision problems also need to be ruled out; for instance, is a person apparently not paying attention to a conversation because they have ADHD, or do they simply have trouble hearing what the other person is saying? Issues of relative maturity also need to be considered, particularly with children, since an elementary school classroom could conceivably include children born almost a year apart, and expecting a younger child to display the same level of maturity than one a year older may not be reasonable. Even if children are approximately the same age, their levels of maturity may be quite different, although those differences typically resolve long before they reach adulthood. When two or more conditions exist in the same person, they are known in medicine as comorbidities ("co" meaning "together" and "morbidities" meaning illnesses), and any treatment plan needs to be personalized to take into account all of an individual's comorbidities and life circumstances.

3

Diagnosing and Managing ADHD

20. How is ADHD diagnosed?

There is no single test to determine if someone has ADHD, and the process of reaching a diagnosis is complex. In part, this is because many of the symptoms associated with ADHD also occur with other conditions, and some behaviors associated with ADHD are also exhibited by people who are considered to be functioning normally. A diagnosis of ADHD must be made by a medical provider (usually a physician, psychiatrist, or licensed psychologist) and typically involves consideration of multiple sources of information, including direct observation of the individual seeking the diagnosis, interviews with the individual and possibly others such as family members, and test results. If the individual being evaluated is a child, the parents or caregivers will almost certainly provide information, as may professionals from the child's school. The purpose of all this information gathering is to gain a clear picture of how the individual is functioning, what problems they are experiencing (both from their own point of view and from that of others around them), how they respond to different environments, and so on. Gathering information from multiple sources can also help the person making the diagnosis determine if the individual's symptoms are caused by ADHD or one of several related conditions, including autism spectrum disorder, and to determine if the individual is experiencing several conditions (comorbidities) simultaneously that could be aided by treatment.

In the United States, the guidelines for ADHD diagnosis are contained within the *Diagnostic and Statistical Manual*, 5th edition (*DSM-5*) published by the American Psychiatric Association. The *DSM* criteria may seem overly specific and technical, but that level of detail is required because human behavior exists on a continuum, yet diagnoses are discrete: a person is diagnosed with ADHD or they are not. The detailed rules and criteria are necessary in order to allow the physician or psychologist to evaluate a varied collection of symptoms and behaviors and link it with one or more conditions, while eliminating other possibilities that may be similar. Fortunately, patients, parents, and teachers do not need to be experts in ADHD diagnosis—that's why evaluations for ADHD are made by medical or psychological professionals.

An ADHD diagnosis requires that an individual show a persistent pattern of inattention or hyperactivity and impulsivity, or a combination, at a level that interferes with their functioning or development. To meet the criteria for inattention, children up to age 16 must display six or more symptoms of inattention that have been present for at least 6 months and are inappropriate for the child's developmental level. For adults and adolescents aged 17 or older, five or more symptoms are required for a diagnosis. Examples of inattention behaviors (more are listed in *DSM-5*) include being easily distracted, being frequently forgetful, having trouble following directions, and losing common and necessary items (e.g., eyeglasses, keys, schoolbooks).

The criteria for a diagnosis of hyperactivity-impulsivity are similar, although the specific behaviors involved are different. Children up to age 16 must show six or more symptoms of hyperactivity-impulsivity, while adults and adolescents age 17 or older need to show five or more. In both cases, the symptoms must have been present for at least 6 months, disrupt the person's functioning, and be inappropriate for their level of development. Examples of hyperactive behavior include frequent fidgeting, leaving one's seat when inappropriate, talking excessively, interrupting others in conversation, and experiencing difficulty in activities that require waiting your turn. The individual, whether child or adolescent or adult, must also have had inattentive-hyperactive symptoms before age 12, and at least some of the symptoms must occur in more than one setting (e.g., both at school and at home, or when interacting with both peers and authority figures).

There are three types of ADHD diagnoses. Combined presentation is a diagnosis signifying that both inattentive and hyperactive-impulsive symptoms have been present for the past six months. A predominantly inattentive presentation diagnosis is returned if only the criteria for the inattentive diagnosis is met, and a predominantly hyperactive-impulsive presentation if only the criteria for hyperactivity-impulsivity are met. A diagnosis may be revised if the individual's symptoms change, and the term "predominantly" in the second and third diagnoses means that symptoms of both types may be present in a person, but only one type occurs at the level required for a diagnosis.

21. What are some common drug treatments for ADHD?

Often a management plan for ADHD includes the use of one or more medications. There has been controversy in the past regarding the use of medications to treat ADHD, and in some cases medications may have been overused to the detriment of the individual being treated. Such abuses should not be allowed to obscure the fact that, for some people with ADHD, the most effective treatment plan may include one or more prescription drugs. Because the response to any medication may vary from one person to the next, the use of medications requires monitoring; it may take some time to find the best medication(s) and dosage(s) for an individual. Finding the right treatment for ADHD is not as simple as, say, prescribing an antibiotic to treat strep throat, and the patient and doctor (and the patient's parents in the case of a child) must work together to find what works best for a particular individual. The use of medications does not preclude other treatments, such as counseling, environmental modification, and neurofeedback, and the goal should always be to create a comprehensive treatment plan tailored to the individual and his or her specific symptoms and circumstances.

The most common medications used to manage ADHD in children and adolescents are stimulants which enhance activity in the prefrontal cortex, a region of the brain which plays an important role in cognitive functions including the regulation of attention, behavior, and emotion. Examples of tasks which draw on the prefrontal cortex include planning and organizing for the future, shifting attention from task to task when required, sustaining attention and concentration in situations when doing so is not immediately rewarding (e.g., listening to a boring lecture), and inhibiting response to internal and external distractions (for instance, ignoring irrelevant stimuli). The logic behind using stimulants to manage ADHD is that people with ADHD often experience deficits in the tasks regulated by the prefrontal cortex, so stimulating it should produce increased activity in that area and thus reduced deficits in those tasks. Studies have found that about 80 percent of children with ADHD experience improved functioning and a reduction in their symptoms when treated with an appropriate stimulant at an effective dosage, which offers cause for optimism but also cautions that it may take some time to find a drug or combination of drugs that will work for a given individual, and to find the right dosage(s). An additional caution is that some prescription stimulant drugs are treated by law as controlled substances which offer the potential for abuse, and any misuse of these drugs can carry criminal penalties, so it is particularly important to take the drugs as prescribed and not allow anyone else to use them.

The most common stimulant drugs used to treat ADHD are preparations of methylphenidate or amphetamine, both of which boost neurotransmission of norepinephrine (noradrenaline) and dopamine in the prefrontal cortex. Common brand names for these drugs include Ritalin (methylphenidate), Methylin (methylphenidate), Focalin (dexmethylphenidate), Adderall (amphetamine), Evekeo (amphetamine), and Dexedrine (dextroamphetamine). Individuals taking prescribed stimulants require clinical monitoring, particularly at the beginning of the treatment, in order to adjust the dosage to the optimal level and to take note of any adverse effects the individual may be experiencing. Certain medical conditions preclude the use of stimulants or require particularly careful monitoring due to possible complications; these conditions include cardiovascular disease, hyperthyroidism, seizure disorders, and hypertension. Stimulant use may also be contraindicated, or require closer than usual monitoring, if the individual is taking certain other drugs, including MAOIs (monoamine oxidase inhibitors), anticoagulant medications, tricyclic antidepressants, and anticonvulsive drugs.

Several nonstimulant medications are also used to treat ADHD and may prove particularly useful for people who do not response to stimulant medications. Atomoxetine, sold under the brand name Strattera, increases the concentration of norepinephrine and dopamine in the prefrontal cortex by inhibiting norepinephrine reuptake. One advantage of atomoxetine over stimulant drugs is that it does not offer the potential for abuse; one disadvantage is that patient response may be slower than with stimulant drugs. Another issue with atomoxetine is that the FDA has determined that it is associated with increased suicidal ideation (although not suicidality) in children and adolescents, so any child or adolescent taking it should be monitored for mood and behavior change and thoughts of self-harm or suicide. Clonidine, sold under the brand name Kapvay, and guanfacine, sold under the brand name Intuniv, are alpha-2 agonists that have helped some individuals with ADHD to regulate attention, impulsivity, and hyperactivity.

Treatment plans for adults with ADHD may include multiple facets, including both psychosocial treatments (e.g., cognitive-behavioral therapy) and medications. As with children, ADHD medications for adults are commonly grouped into two categories: stimulants and non-stimulant medications. Compounds containing stimulants such as methylphenidate and amphetamine are most commonly used to treat adults with ADHD, with some studies finding that 70 percent to 80 percent of adults with ADHD respond favorably to these drugs. Clinical precautions for adults are similar to those for children, with the additional caution that, given the greater freedom enjoyed by adults, the abuse potential of prescription stimulants must be considered, particularly for adults with a history of substance abuse. Several nonstimulant drugs have also proved useful in treating ADHD in adults, including atomoxetine, the antidepressant bupropion (brand names include Wellbutrin and Zyban), clonidine (brand name Kapvay), the anti-narcoleptic modafinil (brand names include Alertec and Provigil), and tricyclic antidepressants such as desipramine (brand name Norpramin).

22. What are some common side effects of ADHD drugs, and can anything be done about them?

While many individuals with ADHD find that prescription medications help them manage their symptoms, it is also unfortunately true that many drugs have unpleasant or disturbing side effects. A side effect is simply some response caused by a drug beyond the effect the drug is meant to have in treating a particular condition—for instance, a drug that improves concentration in people with ADHD may also cause insomnia or disturbed sleep. Many drugs have side effects, and those prescribed for ADHD are no exception, although such side effects are usually mild and may resolve with time. Anyone experiencing side effects from a medication should discuss the matter with their physician, because it may be possible to adjust the dosage or switch to an alternative drug that is effective in treating ADHD but doesn't cause the side effects. There may also be ways for the patient to manage the side effects so they are less unpleasant and cause less interference in the patient's life.

Many of the drugs used to manage ADHD are stimulants which increase the levels of the neurotransmitters dopamine and norepinephrine in the individual's brain, enhancing arousal in the prefrontal cortex. These drugs can make it easier for a person with ADHD to control their attention, thought processes, and motivation, and to reduce their impulsive behavior. The most common stimulants used to treat ADHD include forms of amphetamine or methylphenidate, and either type of drug may be prescribed in a short-acting (immediate release) or long-acting (extended release) form. In general, the effects of short-acting drugs last for four hours or less, while those of long-acting drugs may last as long as 8 or 16 hours. Examples of brand-name ADHD medications and their active ingredient include Ritalin (methylphenidate), Methylin (methylphenidate), Focalin (dexmethylphenidate), Adderall (amphetamine), Dexedrine (dextroamphetamine), Procentra (dextroamphetamine), and Concerta (methylphenidate).

Stimulants can raise the heart rate and systemic blood pressure, although with children and adolescents the increase is usually not enough to cause clinical concern. The average increase in the heart rate due to taking prescribed stimulant medications to treat ADHD is 3–4 beats per minute, and the average increase in blood pressure is 3–4 mmHg (millimeters of mercury) for systolic pressure and 1–2 mmHg for diastolic pressure. However, those figures are averages, and an individual might experience greater increases, to the point where they felt uncomfortable or that their health was impacted. For this reason, it is important to monitor anyone taking stimulants, while anyone taking them who experiences side effects that are unpleasant or interfere with the normal conduct of their life should report that fact to their physician. Other effects experienced by some people taking prescribed stimulants include weight loss, decreased appetite, anxiety, difficulty sleeping, nausea, and involuntary movements (tics). As with changes in heart rate and blood pressure, any patient experiencing these side effects should speak with their physician to see if there is an alternative treatment or a way to manage the side effects.

The medical use of stimulants increases the possibility that the patient may experience a serious cardiac event, such as stroke, myocardial infarction (heart attack), and sudden and unexpected death. While such consequences are rare in children and young adults, and multiple drug trials have shown no significant increase in cardiac effects among young people taking prescribed stimulants, caution is still required when using these drugs. For older adults being treated for ADHD, this risk is higher, and therefore any adult prescribed stimulant drugs should be evaluated for cardiac risk before taking this type of drug and monitored for cardiac complications while taking it. Because cardiac events can be life-threatening, a patient experiencing even relatively mild symptoms suggesting cardiac involvement, such as chest pain or syncope (unexplained fainting or loss of consciousness), should report the matter to their physician immediately.

Several types of nonstimulant medications are also used to treat ADHD. Atomoxetine (brand name Strattera) increases concentration of norepinephrine and dopamine in the prefrontal cortex by inhibiting reuptake of norepinephrine. Atomoxetine should not be used by individuals with liver dysfunction, and individuals taking atomoxetine should be monitored for mood and behavior changes, including increased irritability and thoughts of suicide and self-harm. Common side effects of atomoxetine include nausea, vomiting, diarrhea, fatigue, loss of appetite, and mood swings, although these symptoms often subside over a period of several weeks. Some patients taking atomoxetine also experience insomnia, elevated heart rate, and elevated blood pressure, and any of these symptoms should be discussed with the physician.

Another class of non-stimulant medications used to treat ADHD is alpha-2-agonists, usually in extended-release formulations; examples of this class of drug include clonidine (brand name Kapvay) and guanfacine (brand name Intuniv). Patients should be evaluated for cardiac risk factors and cardiac disease before taking alpha-2-agonists and should have their heart rate and blood pressure monitored. Alpha-2-agonists can worsen depressive symptoms, and thus are not generally used with patients who have a history of depression. Common side effects of clonidine include sedation, dry mouth, headache, dizziness, and constipation, while common side effects of guanfacine include fatigue, rapid heart rate, lower blood pressure, and drowsiness.

23. Are there any foods that can interfere with ADHD treatments?

People taking drugs prescribed to treat ADHD may have heard conflicting reports about interactions between food and ADHD medications. Examining the complex relationships between food and any drug can be challenging because there can be so many factors in play, and because the experiences of one individual may be different from that of another. For any ADHD patient, the individual's physician should be the primary source of information, and any instructions provided by that physician regarding food and medication should be followed, including the timing of taking the medication in relation to eating, and particular foods to avoid while taking the medication. The information in this section is provided as an overview of what is currently known about interactions between food and ADHD drugs but does not constitute medical advice. As always, any difficulties regarding apparent interactions between food and medication should be discussed with the individual's physician, because reactions to food can differ among people.

There are some commonalities in terms of food and medication interaction which have been reported in clinical research, and knowing about these results may be useful to some with ADHD, or the parent of a child with ADHD. It is usually advised that patients taking short-acting methylphenidate-containing medicines (including brand names such as Ritalin and Concerta) be taken on an empty stomach, and that the patient wait 45 minutes to an hour between taking their medication and eating in other to allow the medication to be absorbed. There is also some evidence that consuming a high-fat meal before taking drugs containing drugs amphetamine or dextroamphetamine (including brand names such as Adderall and Dexedrine) can impair absorption of the active ingredient, and thus this pattern of consumption should be avoided.

Acidic foods and foods high in vitamin C, such as orange juice and other citrus fruit products, have also been shown to impair the absorption of drugs containing amphetamine, at least in some individuals. For this reason, patients are often advised to not consume such foods within an hour of taking amphetamine-containing drugs (i.e., avoid acidic foods for one hour before and after taking the drug). High-fat foods can impair the absorption of guanfacine, while other types of food do not, so anyone taking a drug containing guanfacine (such as the brand name drug Intuniv) should not consume high-fat foods for an hour before or after taking the drug. In addition, some physicians advise limiting or eliminating caffeine while taking drugs for ADHD, because caffeine can raise the heart rate and cause an individual to feel restless. Foods containing caffeine include coffee, tea, and some types of soda (this information will be listed on the food label).

Patients taking extended-release medications may be particularly concerned with the possible interactions between their medications and food consumption. Extended-release medications are often taken once per day, usually in the morning, so the timing of the drug with the consumption of breakfast and the foods included in that breakfast are of particular concern. For extended-release drugs containing amphetamine, such as Adderall, consumption of a high-fat breakfast has been shown to reduce drug concentration in the bloodstream for up to 8 hours, potentially reducing the drug's effectiveness. No such effects were found for extended-release drugs containing methylphenidate (such as Concerta): drug concentrations in the bloodstream were not affected by consumption of a high-fat breakfast.

24. Why are stimulants used to treat a condition that has "hyperactivity" in its name?

ADHD is an acronym for "Attention Deficit Hyperactivity Disorder." It may seem surprising that stimulants such as amphetamine are often used to treat a condition that has the word "hyperactivity" (meaning "too much activity," or more specifically too much activity given usual expectations in a particular context) in its name. However, this apparent paradox disappears once you understand what prescribed stimulants can do to help people with ADHD: they are not meant to increase an individual's overall level of activity but to increase activity in a particular part of the brain that is involved in many of the activities that may cause trouble to people with ADHD. While every person with ADHD is unique, and treatment plans should be individualized based on the particular patient and their circumstances, years of clinical research has demonstrated that some people with ADHD are helped by drugs containing stimulants. For those individuals, taking stimulant drugs as prescribed can help them manage their symptoms and function effectively in their lives.

The most common prescription stimulant medications prescribed for ADHD contain amphetamine and methylphenidate, or related substances such as lisdexamfetamine or dexmethylphenidate. Examples of brand-name drugs containing amphetamine include Adderall, Dexedrine, and Procentra, while brand-name drugs containing methylphenidate include Ritalin, Methylin, and Focalin. These drugs have been shown to enhance arousal in the prefrontal cortex, a part of the brain involved in activities such as problem solving, impulse control, and making and executing plans. Both act by increasing dopamine and norepinephrine neurotransmission in the prefrontal cortex, but by somewhat different mechanisms. Methylphenidate inhibits presynaptic dopamine transporters and also inhibits norepinephrine transporters, in the process increasing the concentration of dopamine in the synaptic cleft and increasing dopaminergic neurotransmission. Amphetamine acts as a pseudo-substrate on dopamine transporter and norepinephrine transporter binding sites, thus inhibiting their activity, and also increases catecholamine release. Both amphetamine and methylphenidate also increase dopamine release.

Although medications containing stimulants have been shown to help many people with ADHD, they are powerful stimulant drugs and should only be used as prescribed and as part of a comprehensive treatment plan supervised by a physician. No drug should be considered a "universal fix" for ADHD, and anyone taking these drugs needs to be screened for potential contraindications (such as risk for cardiac events) and monitored for possible complications (which can include anything from temporary loss of appetite to a serious increase in heart rate or blood pressure). If a medication is not working for an individual, or if it is causing side effects that are troublesome to the individual, this should be reported to the physician or care team. It may be possible to change the dosage, substitute a different drug for the one originally prescribed, ameliorate the side effects, or otherwise modify the treatment plan so it works better for the individual patient.

25. I took my friend's ADHD medication and did really well on an exam—does that mean I have ADHD?

Because ADHD medications have been shown to improve cognitive performance and result in better grades or improve work accomplishments for some people with ADHD, it's natural to wonder if they might not also enhance the cognitive performance of people who do not have ADHD. After all, many students, particularly adults and those nearing adulthood, consume caffeine while studying, often in the form of coffee, tea, or energy drinks. They may feel that their performance is improved by the caffeine, not only in the obvious sense of being able to stay awake later and thus have more time to study but also in terms of improved focus and concentration.

Adults who are not students also use caffeine for this purpose, and few would criticize them on this score. In fact, the image of an office worker toiling late at night on some project in order to meet an impending deadline would hardly be complete had they not a cup of coffee or tea close at hand. Such an image is often taken as proof that a person is a hard worker and a dedicated employee, not that they are overworked or are misusing caffeine to stay awake longer than they should. Caffeine is a strong stimulant, and one which is readily available, commonly consumed, and whose use does not incur a social stigma in most contexts. Understanding this societal attitude toward one stimulant makes it easy to see how someone might think that if caffeine is good, prescription medications containing stimulants such as amphetamine might be even better when it comes to increasing an individual's ability to stay awake, keep working, and focus, and thus to perform better on whatever cognitive task is at hand.

We live in a competitive society, and many people face pressures, from a student who wants to get good grades and high test scores to working adults who may feel the need to outcompete their peers or complete high volumes of work in order to win a promotion or just keep their job. Given this context, it's not surprising that some people, despite not having a diagnosis of ADHD or a prescription for ADHD drugs, may try taking stimulants meant to treat ADHD to help them meet these challenges. Stories abound of students facing a tough academic load or an impending high-stakes test who "borrowed" ADHD medications prescribed to their friends, and drugs like Adderall (which contains amphetamine) have been informally referred to as "study drugs" for this reason. This type of use, in which an individual takes a prescription drug which was not prescribed to them, and does so without medical supervision, is entirely distinct from that of a person who takes drugs prescribed for them and is under the care of a physician who can monitor the drug's effects on the individual.

Taking prescription medications not prescribed for you is categorized in the United States as "prescription drug misuse" and has been studied by medical and scientific researchers. As with any illicit behavior, it's difficult to know the extent of prescription drug misuse, because most studies rely on self-reporting, and people are understandably reluctant to reveal that they are engaging in illegal or societally disapproved behaviors. Researchers trying to ascertain how common are behaviors such as underage drinking or cheating on exams face similar challenges—they know self-reporting is probably not accurate, but they don't know how inaccurate it is. Results of surveys regarding self-reported behaviors must therefore be interpreted with caution, and with the understanding that the illicit behavior(s) under study may be far more common than was indicated on the survey.

Given this context, it is also not surprising that different surveys produce different estimates of how common the misuse of prescription drugs is, either nationally or within any subgroup. However imperfect the data may be, recent surveys have indicated that the misuse of prescription drugs is not uncommon in the United States, and that ADHD drugs are among those commonly misused. Nailing down how commonly ADHD drugs are misused has another complication, because many surveys gather data about categories of drugs, not the specific condition they are meant to treat. This means questions are typically phrased to ask about the misuse of "prescription stimulants" rather than about "drugs prescribed for ADHD," and one must extrapolate what percentage of the prescription stimulant misuse referred to drugs commonly used to treat ADHD.

A recent report by the National Institution on Drug Abuse reveals a range of estimates on the extent of misuse of prescription stimulant drugs in the United States. The 2021 National Survey on Drug Use and Health found that about 1.3 percent of respondents over the age of 12 reported misusing prescription stimulants in the past 12 months, which would equate to about 3.7 million people. The same survey found that 0.5 percent of people aged 12 or older had a prescription stimulant use disorder in the past 12 months, which would equate to about 1.5 million people.

Looking at students in middle school and high school, a more specific breakdown is available from the 2022 Monitoring the Future survey. This survey is conducted with students in the eighth, tenth, and twelfth grades, and includes longitudinal follow-up surveys of some high school graduates who participated in previous surveys. This survey found that 3.2 percent of students in eighth grade, 2.1 percent of students in tenth grade, and 2.9 percent of students in twelfth grade reported misusing amphetamines in the past 12 months. Looking at more specific stimulant drugs, 0.7 percent of students in eighth grade, 0.7 percent of students in tenth grade, and 1.1 percent of students in twelfth grade reported misusing Ritalin in the past 12 months. For Adderall, another popular brand-name ADHD drug, the comparable percentages were 2.3 percent, 2.9 percent, and 3.4 percent.

The need to do well in school doesn't end with high school graduation, of course. Medical school is a prime example of a situation in which students are under time pressure and must do well at a challenging sequence of classes and exams in order to achieve their goals. A systematic review of the research literature by Noorine Plumber and colleagues found a wide range of reported use of stimulants, including prescription drugs, among medical school students. The details of the questions asked varied from one survey to another, and it should always be kept in mind that cultural differences among students in different countries could result in different levels of reporting that may not reflect actual differences in the use of nonprescribed stimulants. Across thirteen studies conducted in nine different countries, including the United States and several European and Middle Eastern countries, most found reported use of nonprescribed stimulant medications by medical students in the range of 5 percent to 15 percent. The highest reported use of prescription stimulants found was 47.4 percent, although it should be borne in mind that the sample size for that study was relatively small in relation to the other studies (meaning the results may be less precise), and that the study did not differentiate between prescribed and nonprescribed use of the medications in question.

Although the widespread misuse of ADHD drugs as study and concentration aids might seem to confirm that they are effective when used in this way for people not diagnosed with ADHD, evidence from scientific research is equivocal about the benefits thus gained. In addition, the tasks performed by subjects in studies are necessarily more limited than what is required of a student in a real class or on a real exam, so the results may not apply perfectly to real tasks. Numerous studies of rote-learning tasks, such as recalling lists of paired words, showed no significant improvement in the short term for healthy adults using prescription stimulants as part of the research study (i.e., they were not prescribed to the subjects to treat any condition). Some studies did find improved recall over a longer period, but only with rote tasks and not the kind of complex memory tasks that would be required of a high school or college student. Some studies found that prescription stimulants improved performance on specific creative tasks, and other studies have found improvement in working memory or cognitive control, but in all three cases the improvement was greatest among those with low baseline performance. One possible interpretation of this result is that the drugs may be making up for a deficit in the individuals they help, rather than improving the performance of people already functioning at a high level.

26. What are some common behavioral treatments for ADHD?

While most people are familiar with the idea of treating ADHD with prescription drugs, often behavioral therapies are used in addition to, or instead of, prescription drugs. This is not surprising, because many mental and psychological conditions respond best to a combination of drug and behavioral therapies, and the goal in every case is to find the treatment or combination of treatments that works best for a specific individual. As with any course of treatment, the patient and/or patient's parents should communicate regularly with the medical professional or medical team and keep them informed about whether a therapy is helping or not, because there are many treatment options available.

For children with ADHD, the American Academy of Pediatrics recommends that the first choice of treatment for those younger than 6 should be parental training in behavior management. For children between 6 and 12, the first recommendation for treatment is parental training in behavior management plus drug therapy, and for children over 12, behavior management for the ADHD patient plus drug therapy. These recommendations reflect the increasing ability of older children to learn to manage their behavior: when they are very young, most of the responsibility is placed on the parents, but by the time they reach adolescence, most of the responsibility is placed on the child. No matter who is receiving the behavior therapy training, the goal is to learn positive behaviors and strengthen those already learned while lessening or eliminating unwanted behaviors. For children attending school, the classroom teacher and other educational specialists can also be involved in the behavior therapy, with more of the responsibility shifting from adult to child as the child matures, in the same way that it shifts from parent to child.

Parents enrolling in parent behavioral therapy typically have eight to twelve sessions with the therapist, which may be individual, group (with other parents), or a combination of both. The goal of the sessions is to teach parents strategies to influence their children's behavior. The parents are then expected to practice the strategies between sessions and discuss the success or failure of the program with the therapist in later sessions. Goals of the therapy include teaching parents positive ways to interact with their children and teaching skills and strategies parents can use to manage their child's behavior using structure, positive reinforcement, and consistent discipline. For instance, parents can learn helpful ways to respond when their children are engaging in hyperactive behaviors. They can also teach their children strategies to improve their ability to make and carry out plans, manage their school work, and carry out instructions. Some of the latter strategies are as simple as using planners and checklists consistently, but such basic interventions often make a huge difference in school success and enjoyment for a child who has difficult with executive function.

For adolescents and adults, the emphasis in behavioral training shifts to the person with ADHD, who is mature enough to take more responsibility for their behavior. Older children and adults can learn to recognize the situations in which they struggle, identify "triggers" that may provoke an unwanted response, and can learn and practice positive behaviors to use in triggering situations. As with children, learning and consistently using tools like planners and checklists may be extremely helpful to adolescents and adults with ADHD, who may require more structure than the average person in order to succeed in their studies or at their job. Time management skills can also be taught, as can self-monitoring, so the individual with ADHD can recognize when their first-choice way of approaching their classes or job is not effective, and to switch to a more effective strategy.

27. Are there any alternative medicine treatments that can help with ADHD?

Complementary and alternative medicine (CAM), which includes a broad variety of treatments considered outside the norm of Western medicine, is increasingly being used alongside or in place of more familiar treatments like prescription drugs and behavioral interventions for many conditions. Examples of CAM include dietary interventions, acupuncture, herbal medicines, nutritional supplements, and mind-body practices such as yoga, tai chi, and meditation. While many CAM treatments are available without the consultation of a physician, it is always wise to inform the physician or medical team if using any of these practices, particularly those involving dietary changes, supplements, or herbal medicines, because some of those treatments may interact with the prescribed medical treatment. Many physicians are becoming more knowledgeable about CAM, so it never hurts to ask if the physician has any recommendations regarding CAM treatments that might help an ADHD patient.

Dietary interventions and their usefulness in ADHD are discussed in question 16. In addition to those strategies, some researchers have proposed using nutritional supplements to help treat ADHD. The logic behind this approach is that mineral deficiencies have been identified in children with ADHD in many countries, including the United States, which raises the question of whether taking mineral supplements, primarily zinc and iron, might help lessen ADHD symptoms. Unfortunately, this research is in the early stages, and in some cases has been studied only in animal models, and in others with only small groups of patients, so it can't be said definitively if mineral supplementation will or won't help ADHD patients. On the other hand, the risk of taking appropriate doses of mineral supplements is small (many people do this every day when they take a multivitamin), so it's a question that might be worth raising with one's physician.

Herbal supplements, also known as phytomedicines (medicines derived from plants), are another type of CAM that may interest some patients with ADHD. Plant-based medicines have been used in traditional health systems around the world, and many plants include bioactive compounds that can influence human health. In fact, some common modern pharmaceutical medicines are derived from, or imitations of, substances naturally occurring in plants; examples include aspirin, digoxin, and morphine. However, phytomedicine today tends to focus on the effectiveness of using extracts from the entire plant, rather than isolating a single substance which can be replicated in the lab, because the effectiveness of the plant as medicine may be based on interactions among the many different substances contained in the plant.

In vitro studies (lab studies, literally "done in the glass" rather than with living organisms) of *Rhodiola rosea* (sometimes called "golden root" or "arctic root") has been shown to raise levels of dopamine, serotonin, and norepinephrine. It has also been shown to stimulate the reticular activating system while preventing excess release of the stress hormone cortisol, suggesting that it might be useful in treating ADHD. In human trials, it has been shown to improve cognitive functions, including attention, memory, and accuracy, further suggesting it might help people with ADHD. However, research with this plant is still in the early stages, so the results are more suggestive than definitive. Anyone interested in trying *Rhodiola rosea* to relieve ADHD symptoms should do so under physician supervision to determine the correct dose and to prevent any unintended interaction with other medications.

Ginkgo biloba (which comes from the leaves of the ginkgo or maidenhair tree) has been used for centuries in traditional Chinese medicine to treat memory and cognitive impairments. In vitro and animal studies have found that extract of *Ginkgo biloba* has anti-oxidant properties, inhibits MAO activity, and increases dopamine levels in the prefrontal cortex. Clinical studies with humans have indicated that *Ginkgo biloba* extract can improve attention, memory, fluid intelligence, and processing speed, as compared to a placebo, which suggests it might help people with ADHD. Unfortunately, only a few small trials have been conducted with ADHD patients and *Ginkgo biloba* extract, and they have produced conflicting results, so no definitive statement can be made on its effectiveness. As with other herbal medicines, anyone interested in using *Ginkgo biloba* extract as part of their treatment plan for ADHD should consult with their physician and be monitored for side effects. *Ginkgo biloba* extract is not recommended for people taking anticoagulants (e.g., heparin, warfarin) and should not be taken for two weeks before a scheduled surgery.

Melatonin is a hormone secreted by the pineal gland in humans and is associated with the sleep and wakefulness cycle. It is also present in animals and plants, and responds to darkness and light, increasing secretion in darkness and inhibiting it in light. This helps to explain why people experiencing difficulty with sleep are often advised to be sure there is no light in their bedroom during sleeping hours, and to avoid exposure to television and other light-emitting screens immediately before their bedtime. Taking a melatonin supplement has helped some people with sleep difficulties, and as many people with ADHD experience insomnia and/or disturbed sleep, it's reasonable to ask if melatonin would help them. Only a few studies have been conducted on the effectiveness of melatonin in improving sleep function for children with ADHD, but those conducted have had found promising results and no major adverse effects. Although melatonin can be purchased without prescription in the United States, its use to treat ADHD should be supervised by a physician. In addition, because supplements are not regulated the way prescription medicines are (i.e., there is no assurance that a melatonin product contains the amount of drug claimed on the label), patients should only use supplements whose quality and dosage have been verified.

Acupuncture is a practice in traditional Chinese medicine that is performed by trained specialists. Lin Ang and colleagues found, in a meta-analysis of fourteen studies involving 1,185 ADHD patients, that using acupuncture in addition to conventional medical treatments had positive effects, including reducing hyperactivity and impulsivity and reducing difficulties with learning and conduct. Using acupuncture alone also resulted in improvements for ADHD patients in terms of reduced hyperactivity and impulsivity and fewer learning problems. However, the study's authors note that the potential of bias was high for a number of the studies included in the meta-analysis, so further research with better controls is required before endorsing acupuncture as a treatment for ADHD. It is also worth noting that most of the studies were conducted in China, where acupuncture is part of a long-standing medical tradition that is believed by many to be valid treatment. In the United States, where acupuncture is unfamiliar to many people, patients might be less willing to try acupuncture. In addition, the use of acupuncture in a culture where it is not believed to be helpful could result in worse outcomes than observed in China. This latter effect could be considered the placebo effect in reverse—as a patient may see improvement from administration of an inert substance they believe will help them, so they may not be helped by a treatment they believe to be ineffective.

Yoga is a set of practices developed in ancient India, aspects of which have become popular in the United States and many other countries. While yoga as originally developed (and as practiced by some people today) combined physical, mental, and spiritual practices, in the United States "doing yoga" tends to refer primarily to going through a series of physical exercises, perhaps also including relaxation, meditation, or breathing practices. Some studies have found positive results for ADHD patients who took part in a yoga group, with benefits including improved mood, decreased anxiety, and reduced symptoms of ADHD. Practicing yoga is a noninvasive and generally healthful activity that can be used in combination with other drug and behavioral treatments, and there are no serious contraindications to its use if a given patient is interested in trying it, although it may also be wise to discuss it with one's physician.

Mindfulness meditation, a non-religious practice in which people learn to observe whatever is happening in the present moment without judgment, is also becoming popular in the United States. Small studies have found some beneficial effects of mindfulness meditations training and practice in relieving ADHD symptoms, including improved attention and executive function and reduced behavioral problems, but such improvements did not persist in the long term. Other studies of meditation and ADHD have produced equivocal results, and more studies are required to determine if there are sufficient positive effects to recommend mindfulness meditation to people with ADHD. As with yoga, mindfulness meditation is noninvasive and should not conflict with other types of treatment, although it is always a good idea to discuss it with one's physician.

Neurofeedback teaches people to regulate their own neuronal activity with the assistance of recorded EEG (electroencephalography) or HEG (hemoencephalography) information, both of which are records of the electrical activity in their brain. This EEG or HEG information is used to create a computerized training program that teaches patients to self-regulate their brain activity. This type of treatment is relatively new and has only been studied with a few groups of ADHD patients, and the results of those studies have been mixed. However, this is a promising area of research for the future, so it is possible more effective neurofeedback programs will be developed in the future.

28. Is talk therapy useful for ADHD?

Talk therapy, also called psychotherapy, is a type of treatment aimed at helping people recognize troubling thoughts, emotions, and behaviors, and to understand and change them. Talk therapy can be conducted in individual or group sessions and is usually led by a trained mental health professional such as a psychologist, psychiatrist, or licensed clinical social worker. There are many different types of talk therapy, and any of them may be used alone or in conjunction with other treatments for ADHD, including medication. While some types of talk therapy have been shown to help people with ADHD, as with any treatment, it is important to evaluate if a particular type of therapy is working for a particular individual after a reasonable length of time, and to make adjustments as necessary.

Cognitive-behavioral therapy (CBT) is a type of talk therapy often used to help people with ADHD. CBT is based on the concept that people may have learned patterns of thought or behavior that are not helpful to them, and that they are affected by those patterns even if they are not aware of them. CBT therapy helps individuals identify such patterns and change them. For instance, a person who has experienced failure in school may find their mind flooded with negative thoughts ("I'm so stupid," "I can't do math," "I always blow it," etc.) every time they face an academic challenge. These thoughts distract them from concentrating on the task at hand, thus tending to cause more failure while creating a distorted sense of their own capabilities. However, such thoughts are not inevitable, and CBT can teach a person to identify their negative thoughts, recognize them as a distortion of reality, and substitute more accurate and positive thoughts. By doing so, they can concentrate on the work to be done instead of being distracted by fears, anticipating failure, or simply giving up. Learning to interrupt negative thoughts in this way tends to lead to better performance, thus increasing confidence and setting up the person for more success in the future.

CBT can help people with ADHD learn and practice skills that they may struggle with, such as making plans and carrying them out, avoiding procrastination, or dealing with distracting situations. One technique often used in CBT is role-playing, which allows the patient to rehearse a desired behavior in the safe confines of the therapist's office before trying it in the real world. Because CBT requires patients to take an active part in their own treatment, it is used more often with adults and adolescents than with younger children, while younger children more commonly receive treatment mediated through a parent or teacher who has been trained to help the child learn to manage their behavior. A 2022 review of the effectiveness of CBT for adults with ADHD, conducted by Pablo Luis Lopez and colleagues, found evidence that CBT was helpful for adults with ADHD in the short term, as compared to no therapy or other types of therapy. However, this review also noted that none of the studies included long-term follow-up, that there was a wide variety in the outcomes measured from one study to the next, and that much of the evidence provided was of low quality due to risk of bias.

While it is not a type of psychotherapy, ADHD coaching may be considered a type of talk therapy since it involves the person with ADHD talking with a professional to find ways to help them deal with difficulties they are experiencing in their life. ADHD coaching is customized to a specific individual and is based on the specific areas most important to them; common problems addressed include doing well in school, succeeding at work, and improving interpersonal relationships. The coach helps the client identify areas they would like to improve, helps them create strategies and plans to meet their goals, and provides ongoing support through in-person meetings and/or periodic messages and reminders delivered by telephone, text messages, emails, or other means.

29. Does health insurance cover ADHD treatments?

In the United States, given our fragmented system of health insurance, the best answer to the question "will health insurance cover X?" is usually, "it depends." About two-thirds of Americans with health insurance are covered by a private plan, often a group plan obtained through their employer. The remainder of individuals with health insurance have public coverage, including Medicare (a federal program applying primarily to people over 65 and some people with disabilities) and Medicaid (a joint federal and state system applying primarily to low-income people, with coverage varying from one state to the next). While health care plans in general cover a wide variety of treatments for medical and mental health issues, exactly what's covered and to what degree for any particular individual depend on the provisions of the specific plan covering that person.

However, there are a few commonalities among these varied types of health insurance plans. Since 2014, most individual and small group health care plans in the United States must cover treatment for mental health and substance use disorders. Plans sold through the Health Insurance Marketplace are also required to cover mental health and substance use disorders, as must Medicaid Alternative Benefit Plans. In addition, since passage of the Mental Health Parity and Addiction Equality Act of 2008, most health insurance plans are required to offer coverage for mental health conditions comparable to that offered for physical conditions. However, the Mental Health Parity and Addiction Equality Act does not prohibit deductibles, required copayments, or conditions that may make it difficult or impossible for patients to access mental health care, but only specifies that the rules for accessing mental health care cannot be more restrictive than those within the same plan for medical or surgical care.

Even Medicare is not as simple as it seems, because most people covered by it are actually covered by several different plans which exist in multiple versions. Coverage by the basic Medicare plan (Part A) is consistent across the United States but applies primarily to treatment received in a hospital or other care facility. Most people also purchase a supplemental insurance plan (Medicare Part B) which covers outpatient medical and mental health care, and a prescription drug insurance plan (Medicare Part D). In addition, some people are covered by a HMO-style plan known as Medicare Advantage. The services and drugs covered by those plans, and the fees an individual may have to pay to access them, can vary widely from one plan to the next.

Because Medicaid is administered at the state level, the question of who is eligible for coverage, and what that coverage will pay for, varies widely from one state to the next. Different states have different rules regarding accessing care, and the burden is always on the person using Medicaid to inform themselves of the details of the plan applying to them. To take one example, as of 2015 more than half of the state Medicaid programs required prior authorization for prescribed ADHD medication. This means that prescriptions for drugs used to treat ADHD must undergo an extra level of review, usually by being submitted to the state Medicaid office for approval, before they can be filled. A key motivation behind prior authorization is controlling costs, but it also results in additional administrative burden for the prescribing physician and delay in the prescribed medication reaching the person that needs it. If such bureaucratic requirements are sufficiently burdensome, they may effectively prevent some people from receiving care to which they are theoretically entitled. Some states have additional restrictions requiring ADHD care, such as requiring people under age 18 to undergo a psychological evaluation before ADHD medication will be approved.

Because private health insurance plans are offered by many different insurance companies, and even group plans offered by the same insurer may differ from one employer to the next, it's difficult to make general statements about what is and isn't covered, what kinds of copays or coinsurance (fees paid by the user to access services) are required for particular services or drugs, or the procedures the insured person (or the insured person's parents in the case of a child) must follow to get authorization for care. In all cases, however, it is necessary to know the details of your own specific insurance plan and become familiar with their requirements and procedures. Failure to do so could result in the insurance company refusing to pay for care that has already been delivered, leaving the patient with a large and unexpected bill to pay. Rules about coverage, copayments, and so on often change from one year to the next within a plan as well, so it is also necessary to have the most current information about whatever is covered this year by a particular plan.

Fortunately, people covered by private insurance have some protections. Every health insurance company is required to have an internal complaints procedure, so if you believe coverage has been denied in error, going through this internal procedure may resolve the issue. If it does not, the next step is to contact the state insurance commissioner for your state, who may be able to help resolve the problem. A majority of states also have independent review boards that can examine your case and have the ability to overrule the insurance company's decision. There are also many organizations providing support to people with ADHD and the parents of children with ADHD who may be able to provide advice or refer you to others who can help with your case. Unfortunately, the need to go through such procedures adds a burden to people who need to access denied care.

30. Can ADHD be cured?

It used to be believed that ADHD was a condition of childhood, so that children with ADHD would "grow out of it" as they matured and became adults. This model was based on the belief that ADHD could be cured through maturation and may have been based on the observation that the symptoms affecting children with ADHD are less commonly observed in adults. However, today medical researchers believe that ADHD is a lifelong condition, so children with ADHD become adults with ADHD. Therefore, the model for treating ADHD today is not that of infectious disease that is expected to last for only a limited time but of chronic condition that may be present throughout a person's lifetime. A chronic disease is defined as a disease that lasts a year or longer, and which requires ongoing medical attention or imposes some limitations on activities. Many Americans live full and productive lives while dealing with chronic diseases such as arthritis and diabetes, and with appropriate care and education, people with ADHD can also live a life similar to what would have lived without the disease. The focus on ADHD treatment therefore is on meeting the person where they are and helping them understand their condition, control their symptoms, and achieve their goals.

With infectious disease, often the disease-causing agent can be destroyed and cure achieved, as when a person with strep throat takes antibiotics which kill the bacteria causing the disease. In contrast, a person with a chronic disease condition should not expect to be cured but can learn to live with their disease or condition and minimize its negative effects on their life. This approach includes using whatever medical science can offer to help them control their symptoms, so they interfere as little as possible with their life, analogous to the way a diabetic person can learn to manage and control their blood sugar. Given this understanding, the focus of ADHD treatment today is on reducing symptoms that are problematic to the person with ADHD and helping them to function as well as they can in the world, with no expectations that the ADHD will ever go away.

Although ADHD can't be cured, it can be managed so well that, to someone looking in from the outside, it may seem to be cured. As people with ADHD mature, they can become more independent about managing their care and more proactive about identifying situations in which they will function well, while also identifying others which may be less suitable for them. The types of treatment and other support needed by people with ADHD over the years may also change—for instance, a child may take medication and require a lot of support from parents and teachers but the same person may find that as an adult they do need the medication and or any more support than an average person. Or they may find that different drugs or dosages are more helpful than whatever helped them when they were children. The point in all cases is to adjust the treatment and support to the individual to help them thrive.

31. I take prescription medications for ADHD. Will I have to take them for my entire life?

Today we realize that ADHD is best thought of as a condition that can last a lifetime, so children with ADHD become adults with ADHD. However, that doesn't mean that every person with ADHD will require exactly the same treatments over their life span, because as they mature their needs will most likely change. Individualized treatment is the key: the emphasis in ADHD care is therefore on helping each person lead their best life given their age, circumstances, severity of symptoms, and other factors. This means that the treatment most appropriate to any individual with ADHD will probably change multiple times over their life.

Recognition that adults can have ADHD is relatively recent, and there isn't a great deal of longitudinal research into how the needs of a person with ADHD change over a lifetime. However, some research has found that about half of children who take medication for ADHD will also need to take medicine to control their ADHD in adulthood. To look at the same question from the other side, you could say that about half of children who take medication for ADHD do not need to take it in adulthood. But whichever way you look at it, the point is that each person needs to do what is effective for them given their circumstances, including their age, and there should be no stigma for taking drugs to control ADHD at any age.

People may also be concerned about the health implications of taking drugs to treat ADHD for years and years, particularly if that use begins in childhood. Fortunately, the research available indicates that it is safe to take ADHD drugs for years at a time, and the side effects experienced by long-term users of ADHD drugs are mostly mild and manageable, and that result holds for both children and adults. Every person is different, of course, and the physician should always be consulted if a patient is experiencing troublesome side effects of medication, or if the medication seems to be working less effectively than when initially prescribed.

32. What can I do if my prescribed treatment is not working?

ADHD is a complex condition and a treatment that works for one person may not work for the next. Some studies have found that the most common stimulants prescribed to people with ADHD, methylphenidate and amphetamine, fail to work in about 10 percent of patients. In addition, a treatment may become less effective over time, so what once worked for a person is no longer working today. There's no reason to stick with a treatment that is not working, since many different types of treatments are available. If a patient does not experience improvement on one course of treatment (which can include any combination of prescription drugs, behavioral interventions, and psychotherapy), adjustments can be made, and the process can continue until a treatment or combination of treatments is found that does work. Perhaps the drug dosage needs to be changed, perhaps a different drug should be tried, or perhaps a different mode of talk therapy would be more useful. Communication with the physician or care team is crucial because they can't know what is going on with an ADHD patient unless the patient or their parents tells them. The physician or care team can also help the patient and/or parents understand how prescribed drugs or treatments work, and how quickly they should see improvements, so that their expectations are reasonable.

Many factors can be involved in why a treatment is not effective for a particular individual. The most basic reason is that every person is different, with different body chemistry, and so the mechanism of the drug doesn't work for one person as it does for others. This is true of many types of drugs, not only those prescribed for ADHD, and is not a judgment or a criticism of the individual. Instead, it simply indicates that a different drug or combination of therapies should be tried. Life events can also play a role—for instance, if a person is in a new and stressful situation, their symptoms may worsen, and an adjustment to their medication may be necessary to help them function effectively. Other medical conditions can also interact with ADHD, making treatment less effective, including depression and anxiety. These disorders may require treatment independently of the prescribed ADHD treatment. The use of abuse of alcohol and recreational drugs can also interact with ADHD symptoms and treatment, so it is important to speak honestly with your physician about such matters.

33. What is a "drug holiday," and why are they sometimes recommended?

A drug holiday, or planned medicine holiday, is a period of time during which a person stops taking the drugs prescribed for them, by recommendation of their physician and under medical supervision. Drug holidays should not be tried spontaneously by someone taking prescribed medication: instead they should discuss the matter with their physician and remain under medical supervision during the period in which they aren't taking the drug. Simply ceasing to take prescribed drugs, without medical advice or supervision, is a bad idea because there could be harmful effects that the individual might not know how to manage. They are good reasons for drug holidays taken under medical supervision, however: they allow the patient to see how they function without the drug, reduce the possibility that the patient develops a tolerance to the drug (thus reducing the risk that higher doses will be required to produce the same effect), and give the patient a break from any side effects caused by the drugs.

There has been particular concern about the long-term use of methylphenidate (the active ingredient in drugs such as Concerta and Ritalin) by children and adolescents because of the side effects experienced by some that take it, including loss of appetite, insomnia, and reduced gains in height and weight. The benefits gained by controlling ADHD must be balanced against these potential harms, and children and adolescents taking drugs containing methylphenidate should be monitored for side effects and have their medication protocol reviewed at least once a year. This review may include discussion of whether the patient should take a trial period off the drug, under medical supervision, before deciding if the dosage needs to be adjusted or if the drug should be discontinued.

The main risk of taking a drug holiday from prescribed drugs is that the symptoms controlled by the drugs may return in their absence. For this reason, drug holidays should be planned and scheduled to minimize disruption in the life of the patient and/or his or her family. For school-age children and adolescents, often drug holidays are scheduled during the summer break or holidays, because withdrawing ADHD drugs may result in difficulties in concentration and self-control. Both the patient (if old enough to understand) and parents should be informed of what may happen during a drug holiday, the reasons for taking one, and possible symptoms or reactions they need to monitor. As always, treating ADHD is a partnership among the patient, physician, and (for children and adolescents) the parents, and the physician needs to know how any change in treatment is working for the patient. Sometimes a patient does well enough during a drug holiday that they can stop taking the drug entirely, or switch to a lower dosage, and even if they return to taking the same dosage as before, their body may benefit from taking a break from the drug.

4

Living with ADHD

34. Should I tell anyone at my school that I have ADHD?

Many people with ADHD are enrolled in formal education. A student with ADHD, or the parents of a child with ADHD, may wonder if the school should be informed about the student's condition, and, if so, who should receive that information. The answer to this question is specific to each person and may depend on several considerations, including the severity of the ADHD symptoms, the age and maturity level of the student, the preferences of the person with ADHD and/or their parents, the possibility of accessing special services or accommodations that may help them succeed in their education, and the perceived receptiveness and the expected response of school officials to such information. Some schools, particularly at the tertiary (post-high school, e.g., college or university) level, have an office dedicated to assisting students with disabilities, including ADHD. If such an office exists, that is the place to start, because the people working in it can inform the student and/or parents about their rights and the procedures they should follow.

In the United States, two laws protect the educational rights of people with disabilities, including ADHD. Section 504 of the Vocational Rehabilitation Act of 1973 applies to all institutions which receive federal funds (which includes most if not all schools), prohibits discrimination against people with disabilities, and may require school districts to make appropriate accommodations for students with disabilities. It is a civil rights law aimed at preventing discrimination against people who meet any of three requirements: they have a mental or physical impairment that substantially limits their ability to take part in "major life activities," they have a history of having had such an impairment, or they are regarded as having such an impairment (i.e., other people think they have an impairment). Attending school qualifies as a major life activity, so if a person's ADHD symptoms are serious enough that they interfere with a student taking part in education, that student is entitled to accommodations which may include special educational services or variations in procedures such as testing. Persons who meet the second or third but not the first requirement are protected from discrimination under the Act (for instance, a previous diagnosis of ADHD should not in and of itself be used to prevent a student from taking part in school activities or to enroll in specific classes) but are not entitled to special educational services.

The spirit of the Vocational Rehabilitation Act is that each student should receive a free and appropriate education. Being eligible for accommodations and special education services does not mean the student will be placed in separate special education classes—in fact, students protected under Section 504 must be taught in a regular classroom unless it is impossible to meet their needs in that way. Accommodations, such as allowing a student to take exams separately from the class, in a distraction-free environment, are permitted even if the student is otherwise taught alongside other students.

The Individuals with Disabilities Education Act (IDEA) of 1990 specifies that students with qualified disabilities must be provided with special educational services to meet their specific needs. Thirteen categories of disabilities are included in this law, and an individual seeking special services must demonstrate both that they have a condition fitting into one of the thirteen categories and that this condition affects their ability to succeed in school. When IDEA was passed in 1990, ADHD was not included as a protected disability, but it was added as such in 1991, so today schools must provide appropriate education services for students with ADHD. Such students usually qualify for services under one or more of three categories: learning disability, emotional disorder, or other health impairment. The provision of such services begins with an evaluation to determine the student's educational needs (for a minor child, parents must give permission for such an evaluation to be conducted), and the result of that evaluation is used to create a written individualized education program (IEP). Whatever services or accommodations are indicated in the IEP must be provided by the school, and the student or their family cannot be charged for these services, which are considered part of the free and appropriate education to which every American child is entitled.

If a school can't meet the educational needs of an individual student, the student may be enrolled in a private school that can meet their needs, and the school district must pay for it. Because this can be a major expense, school districts have sometimes resisted paying for such a placement, and may claim they are offering appropriate services for a student while the student's parents may feel that they are not. Such a dispute led to a court case in California in 1995 that established the right of IDEA-protected students to attend private school at the expense of their school district if the district schools are not providing them with appropriate educational services. In this case, the student in question was a ninth-grader who was flunking all his classes at his local public high school. His performance did not improve with the special educational provisions set up by the school, so his parents enrolled him in a private school and then sued the school district for the tuition. A federal court ruled that the school district had to pay the student's tuition and also the family's legal fees, and in 1997 IDEA was amended to specify the right of a student to attend private school at the district's expense if particular conditions were met. These conditions are strict, however, and students and families who feel their needs are not being met by the school district should be prepared to take their case to court.

A student with ADHD may be eligible for protection under both IDEA and Section 504. Schools often prefer students seek protection under Section 504, because it protects the student from discrimination but does not require the creation of an IEP or spell out specific categories of disability that must be accommodated. This gives schools more flexibility in meeting a student's needs and requires only that students with disabilities receive an education as adequate to them as do students without disabilities. These differences mean that it may be less expensive for a school or school district to meet their legal obligations under Section 504. In contrast, parents and individuals with ADHD often prefer to seek protection under IDEA, because it is much more specific about what a school must do to meet the needs of a protected student and defines an adequate education as one that meets the needs of a specific individual, rather than simply being as good as that received by other students at the school. Parents may also feel the need to access the provision in IDEA that the school district must pay for the student to receive the services necessary if the school cannot provide them, and there is no corresponding provision in Section 504.

If an individual's symptoms are mild and well controlled, and they are succeeding well in school, they may choose to not seek accommodations or to inform anyone at the school that they have ADHD. This is most likely to occur with older students, particularly those attending college and university, who may feel that professors or fellow students may stigmatize them for having ADHD. They may also choose to keep this information private because they feel that employers and others may hold prejudice against people with ADHD, so that their ability to achieve their goals may be limited not by their ADHD but by prejudice against people with that condition. This may be a reasonable choice for some individuals, as there is no requirement to inform anyone about ADHD or any other medical condition. Because many tertiary institutions have an office dedicated to accessibility, students may choose to register with them. Any information they provide to that office will be kept confidential, and they can choose to disclose to professors and others on a case-by-case basis. For instance, a student might request accommodations for classes that include a lot of mathematics, such as extra time on exams, but not feel the need for any accommodations for classes in the humanities. If the student follows the procedures specified by the school, and provides appropriate documentation, instructors must provide reasonable accommodations when requested and are prohibited from discriminating against students who request such accommodations.

35. What accommodations can be requested for students with ADHD, and how can I request them?

Many types of accommodations can be requested for students with ADHD, and if the student qualifies for protection under either Section 504 of the Vocational Rehabilitation Act of 1973 or the Individuals with Disabilities Education Act (IDEA) of 1990, the school or school district has a legal obligation to meet the student's needs. There are some differences between the two laws—Section 504 is a civil rights law protecting people with disability from discrimination, while IDEA is an education-specific law that spells out in greater detail the rights of the disabled student and the types of services that must be provided, including assessment and creation of an IEP—but many of the most common types of accommodations are covered by both laws. The professional who evaluates the student and determines that they have ADHD and are entitled to accommodations or other special educational services can be asked to specify exactly what is needed in a letter, which can then be shared with the school's accessibility office or whoever is in charge of helping students who need accommodations.

Some requests for accommodations are relatively easily met, and such requests are generally covered by both IDEA and Section 504. For instance, because students with ADHD may have slower mental processing and difficulties in maintaining concentration on a task, they may ask to be allowed to take extra time to complete exams or to take their exams in a private room that is quiet and free of distractions. They may also request to use specific technology to help them complete some tasks, such as using a laptop to take notes in class, even if other students are expected to take notes by hand. Students, particularly younger students, may request that they be allowed regular breaks from instruction and/ or be allowed to move around the classroom at regular intervals. They may request additional materials, such as printed copies of slides, or may ask for permission to record lectures so they can review them later. Any student may request additional assistance in staying organized, for instance, to have access to a professor's PowerPoint slides in advance of lectures, and younger students may request additional feedback to help them stay on track.

A student protected under IDEA can request more specific and far-ranging accommodations as well. Each student qualified under IDEA will have already been evaluated by a professional in order to get their diagnosis. They may require a second evaluation to determine their specific educational needs, and the results of that evaluation will be used to create an IEP, or individual education plan, a written document specifying what services or accommodations are required for them. Examples of the kind of accommodations and assistance that may be mandated under IDEA include special classes, individualized instruction, extra tutoring, psychological services, and assistance with tasks such as note-taking or computer use. If a school cannot meet a student's specific education needs as determined under IDEA, the school or district must pay for the student to receive them elsewhere, even if that means paying the tuition for the student to attend a private school appropriate for them.

36. I'm a student with ADHD—what can I do to help myself excel academically?

The most useful thing anyone with ADHD can do is to understand themselves, their strengths and weaknesses, and to use that information to formulate plans to reach their goals. While it's possible to list some issues that many people with ADHD have encountered with regard to education, and some strategies that have proved successful in dealing with these issues, every person with ADHD is different and ultimately is responsible for managing themselves and their environment as best they can. Of course, with younger students, adults may need to provide more support and guidance, but high school and university students can take a lot of responsibility toward guiding their own success. Above all, it's important for a person with ADHD to understand themselves and their condition and to take a practical approach toward dealing with it, with a focus on doing what is necessary to succeed rather than blaming either oneself or the environment.

If a student has a diagnosis of ADHD, they are entitled to request accommodations in the classroom and in procedures such as test-taking in order to meet their needs. Often schools, particularly at the tertiary level, have a person or office devoted to helping students who require accommodations, and that person or office can be a great ally as the student with ADHD progresses through their education. Examples of accommodations which an ADHD student may request include extra time on exams, a quiet and distraction-free room for taking exams, using technology to help them stay organized and on track, and provision of printed materials such as lecture notes or PowerPoint slides in advance of lectures.

People with ADHD often struggle with organization and planning tasks, and it is perfectly legitimate to use external aids such as a paper planner and/ or digital calendar to keep track of deadlines, quiz and exam dates, and so on. Some people with ADHD find it useful to plan out their entire day on paper, including specific blocks of time to study different subjects, and time to relax and socialize. This may be particularly important in college, when students are expected to be able to organize their own time and set long-terms goals. In truth, people without ADHD often struggle to make the transition, since it is quite a change from high school where the school exerted much greater control over how the student spent their time. It's also important for people with ADHD to be sure they're getting enough sleep and following a generally healthy lifestyle, with nutritious food and sufficient exercise, since the lack of structure in college life makes it easy to neglect those things.

If a student with ADHD is taking medication, it's important that they are aware of how it affects them and their attention. It may be necessary to adjust the timing or dosage of medications to meet the new demands of higher education, and of course this must be done with the assistance of a medical professional. Scheduling classes and other activities should also be done with the characteristics of the individual student in mind—for instance, does the student think more clearly in the morning or the afternoon? Do they need periodic breaks throughout the day to relax and refresh? Should they reduce their course load in order to have the necessary time and energy to succeed in each class? This kind of self-awareness is useful to anyone, so if people with ADHD have to confront these issues more directly than most people, that may serve as an advantage to them in the long run.

Some specific methods of organization have proven useful for many people with ADHD, although of course each individual must try them out to see if they work for them. Interestingly enough, many of these strategies also work well for people without ADHD, so they might be considered useful general planning strategies. One is to break down long assignments such as a term paper into small parts, and to assign due dates to each step. A similar approach can be used to study for exams—rather than trying to review everything at the last minute, assigning dates to review different chapters or topic throughout the semester generally results in better retention of the material.

Self-awareness is the key to successful studying—each person has to know what they need to do to learn the material assigned and do well on exams or other evaluations. The most useful study techniques generally require the student to be active, so quizzing yourself over what you have read is a better strategy than simply rereading or highlighting a passage. In math and science classes, many students find that working many problems, with focus on understanding why they are doing each step, helps them both learn the material of a particular course and come to understand how their own thought processes work. Writing out your own notes and creating flashcards to review key points is also useful for many students, who find that the act of writing itself helps them to absorb and remember the material.

Spacing out study time is a technique that many find useful. One way to do this is through the so-called "pomodoro" technique, in which the student sets a timer and studies for a particular number of minutes (often 20 or 25), then takes a short break (often 5 minutes) before returning to studying. The person who developed this technique used a kitchen timer shaped like a tomato ("pomodoro" means "tomato" in Italian, the native language of the originator), hence the name. In fact, any timing mechanism will work, and there are online study timers that can be set up to suit each individual student, some of which also keep records of the amount of time spend studying on different subjects. Using such a system may not only result in more efficient studying but also help the student understand how much time they need to devote to each class in order to master it.

A final suggestion is to be aware of what you like and what you are good at, and, conversely what you don't like and aren't good at. The social as well as intellectual aspects of majors are important in this regard—if most of the students in a field of study are outgoing and lots of group projects play a major role in the curriculum, that may not be the best choice for someone who is introverted and has difficulty communicating and socializing. On the other hand, people with ADHD often find they have great powers of concentration when they are interested in a subject and can work alone effectively, attributes that are associated with success in fields like science and computer programming. The key point is that the student should choose their direction by considering the typical conditions of work in a field as well as the intellectual requirements they must meet. Finding the right "fit" in terms of major may be more important for people with ADHD than for the student body in general, and so it's worth taking the time to honestly consider that that best fit might be.

37. What are some good career paths for people with ADHD?

A simple internet search will turn up multiple lists of best jobs for people with ADHD, but it's seldom the same list twice. The truth is that each people must determine for themselves which career paths best match their interests and abilities, and that is as true of people with ADHD as of people without it. Such a search may be guided in part by lists compiled by others, but they are only a tool in a search in which the individual must know their own strengths and weaknesses and does their own research to find out what career paths suit them best. Counselors and other advisors can help in this question, and there are various tests and inventories available that may help an individual narrow down their career choices. Of course, no single test is definitive and the results of any test should be discussed with an expert and considered in the light of other types of information as well.

High school and college campuses often have a number of resources available to help students identify career fields of interest. These often include career centers and counselors, and students should not be shy about accessing these resources. Practical experience can also be useful, and many schools can arrange "shadowing" opportunities, where a student spends a day observing a professional in their field of interest, a practice which helps them understand the flow of the work day and the social as well as technical requirements for succeeding in a particular job. Internships can also be useful in testing a career path because they provide a sort of intermediate state between being a student and being a full-time worker, giving the student a chance to learn more about their field of choice and to make contacts within the field. An added bonus with internships is that it allows the intern to demonstrate what they can do, and successful completion of an internship may well lead to a job offer.

Many people with ADHD have a talent and interest for technical fields— math, the sciences, engineering, computer science, and so on. Some people have even called ADHD a "superpower" for success in these fields, because hyperfocus allows them to concentrate intensely on what is needed to solve a particular problem, while other people may get distracted with unimportant details. Success in classwork is often a good indication of talent in these fields: most people find such subjects difficult, while a person with ADHD may find the subjects fairly easy and intuitive. This is not surprising if we remember that ADHD affects brain function. Interest in a particular field is also an indicator that it may be a good match—a student who spends their free time on math puzzles, for instance, may be a good match for any number of technical careers. How comfortable a student feels around their professors and peers may also be a good indication of a career match, because the students of today are the colleagues of tomorrow, and the professors of today can help students determine if a given career field is for them.

STEM (science, technology, engineering, math) fields, which offer objective means to evaluate one's work, may also be a good fit for people with ADHD who don't come off well in general job interviews but do very well when solving specific problems under pressure. For the same reason, STEM fields are often a good fit for people who are less interested in, or less skilled at, the social interactions that form a large part of some jobs. Being highly skilled in a technical field few people understand can provide a kind of "insulation" that protects the worker from criticism due to their social shortcomings, and people with ADHD often feel more comfortable being evaluated based on the quality of their work rather than how others perceive them.

Some people with ADHD find they relate better to children and young people than to adults. For such individuals, a career in teaching, child social work, or child psychology may be a good match. Others may discover they have a gift for working with words and may be a good match for careers involving writing and editing, including technical writing, which requires talent in both scientific fields and writing. Some find they work best by themselves and prefer taking on the risk and making all the decisions to working as part of a team, in which case focusing on entrepreneurship and running one's own business may be the best choice. Some find they do well under stress and can make decisions quickly and efficiently, in which case a job like an emergency-room physician or emergency medical technician may be a good fit. For people who are bored with routine, a job in which each day is different, as is the case for emergency responders, may be a better fit than a more conventional job (e.g., working in an office or a store) in which one day is very much like the next.

People with ADHD often have creative ideas and show a strong ability to think outside the box—in other words, to think of new ways to do things that may be completely different from the general practice. While this can be a valuable talent, leading to important breakthroughs, it's not appreciated in every work situation, and may even be considered disruptive. A mismatch between the abilities of a worker with ADHD and the expectations of the workplace may be one reason people with ADHD change jobs more frequently than those without it, and a person with ADHD may not be aware that this mismatch is the reason they are having difficulties. A counselor or other professional can help people with ADHD identify why they may be experiencing conflict in their workplace, despite their best efforts to succeed, and suggest ways to deal with the conflict or to find a new job that is a better fit.

There have not been a lot of research into what kind of work adults with ADHD do, how they feel about their jobs, or what factors they think are important to succeed. In fact, no national representative survey has been conducted on the order of the health surveys conducted by the CDC and other federal agencies on a regular basis. However, *ADDitude* magazine did conduct a poll in 2023 with over 1,450 adults with ADHD, and while these results can't be generalized to the ADHD adult population (because we don't know how the sample was drawn or how the characteristics of the respondents relate to the entire population of adults with ADHD), they do provide suggestive insights and directions for future research.

Encouragingly, most of the respondents to the *ADDitude* poll were leading what they considered to be happy and successful lives, and enjoyed and took pride in their work. Over two-thirds had completed at least an undergraduate degree, and more than half were earning above the US median income. They worked in a variety of industries, with almost half in health care or education, and smaller numbers in government, technology, sales, or legal professions. Respondents indicated the characteristics they sought in jobs, which include variety, the chance to be creative and solve problems, having a sense of purpose on the job, having the ability to keep learning new things, and being able to move around and maintain a sense of independence.

At the same time, many respondents mentioned the challenges they faced related to their ADHD and indicated that it was important for the individual worker to find ways to work around these difficulties. Most said they had not asked for formal workplace accommodations, but devised ways to solve these problems on their own. The most common issue cited by respondents was distractibility, followed by difficulty managing time, disorganization, problems with working memory, and boredom, each of which was mentioned by at least 50 percent of respondents. Other issues named by respondents included heightened emotionality, impulsivity, social challenges, and high energy.

38. Should I tell my employer I have ADHD?

The employment rights of people with ADHD are protected under several laws, but the question of whether to mention to an employer that one has ADHD is a question that each individual must answer for themselves. The truth is that many decisions regard matters like promotion are partly subjective, and some people hold a prejudice against people with ADHD. Understanding this, the employee must weigh what they hope to gain by disclosing and/or asking for accommodations against what they might lose. There is no obligation to disclose, and even with legal protections in place, it's natural to worry if disclosure might lead to discrimination in terms of hiring, promotion, or work assignments. After all, in a competitive job market with many well-qualified applicants, it's often impossible to establish why one person was chosen and others were not. Similarly, in a workplace with many capable and hardworking employees, the number of people qualified for promotion probably exceeds the number of promotions available, and minor factors could have enough influence that one person is chosen over another.

Many people, including employers and supervisors, don't understand ADHD and how it may affect someone's ability to function. Lacking that understanding, they may simply resent an employee who asks for accommodations, thinking it to be akin to asking for special privileges or seeking to be the center of attention. This attitude is wrong but not uncommon, and proving discrimination in court can be difficult and costly. In addition, an employee who does receive accommodations may be privately labeled in some people's minds as a troublemaker, and some people may prefer to simply avoid working with them, making it difficult for the person with ADHD to be integrated into the work environment.

Given this context, it may be wise to not disclose if you are doing well on the job and don't need any accommodations other than what you can provide for yourself. On the other hand, if you are having trouble at work, or are about to be fired, then action is required and it might be wise to seek accommodations. While we don't know a lot about how people with ADHD function on the job, because the topic has not been well studied, we do know from one poll conducted in 2023 by *ADDitude* magazine that many working adults with ADHD have chosen to not ask for accommodations, but to find their own workarounds to issues they experienced. Granted, this poll may not be representative of adults with ADHD in general, because the respondents had relatively high incomes and levels of education and were largely happy with their jobs. However, it is useful to know that many adults with ADHD are not unemployed or struggling at work, and that relatively simple adaptations were enough to allow at least some people with ADHD to succeed. Many of the workarounds named in the poll are also used by people without ADHD—for instance, wearing headphones to limit distractibility from office noise, using planners and other scheduling aids to manage time, writing notes to avoid burdening their short-term memory, and dividing long-term tasks into a number of short-term goals to provide a sense of structure and accomplishment in the work day. The key is to find a system that works for you, and that is compatible with your workplace, and to use it consistently.

If an employee with ADHD does choose to seek accommodations, or feels they have been discriminated against, their rights are protected under two federal laws which prohibit discrimination against people with disabilities: The Rehabilitation Act of 1973 (RA) and the Americans with Disabilities Act of 1990 (ADA), the latter including the ADA Amendments Act of 2008 (ADAAA). A third law which might offer protection is the Family and Medical Leave Act (FMLA), which allows some employees the right to take 12 weeks of unpaid leave under certain circumstances, including the inability to work due to a serious health condition, which might include ADHD. Some states offer additional protections beyond what these two laws offer, and the employee with ADHD should consult with a lawyer or other legal advisor to see exactly what protections apply to their situation. Usually an official diagnosis of ADHD is required to seek accommodations, but there could be exceptions depending on the circumstances also.

If an employee does decide to seek accommodations, this can be framed in a positive manner that emphasizes their strengths and the benefits to the company of providing the accommodations, rather than going immediately to legal threats or focusing on their weaknesses. After all, employers are interested in what will benefit them, so stating requests in terms of what the employee brings to the company, and how they could do their work even better with a small accommodation, are more likely to meet with a positive response and also to foster a good working relationship for the future.

39. What are some tips to help people with ADHD thrive in the workplace?

In order to succeed at work, people with ADHD need to know themselves, be honest about their strengths and weaknesses, and carefully consider the kind of working environment they prefer. These issues apply to people without

ADHD as well, but they are of additional importance for people with ADHD since most workplaces are not designed with their needs in mind. For instance, a level of ambient noise that is considered normal by most people might prove distracting to a person with ADHD, and if the person with ADHD can work out an accommodation that allows them to thrive, that may be the best solution for everyone. A workplace is in part a social environment, and if one person is constantly making demands that require other people to change their behavior to accommodate that person's needs, the understandable response may be resentment, which can damage working relationships in the future.

The most common workplace challenges for people with ADHD include distractibility, excess activity, memory issues, planning and time management, and interpersonal interactions. Fortunately, these challenges can sometimes be met with simple adjustments that are used by people without ADHD as well, and that don't require disclosure or demanding that anyone else change their behavior.

Many people with ADHD find they are more distractible than the average adult, and this can interfere with their ability to concentrate on their work and complete tasks in a timely fashion. To deal with external distractions, such as noise or movement, the individual could try using headphones and/or requesting a desk in a part of the office with less foot traffic. It may be possible to create physical barriers as well, such as adding cubicle dividers to a desk, if that is permitted in the office. Many people with ADHD are also prone to internal distractions and may find themselves wasting time on social media rather than doing their work. Apps are available to track how much time is spent on different websites, and it is also possible to lock oneself out of some websites during the work day. Self-awareness can also help in dealing with distractions—for instance, when tempted to go on a social media website, a person could instead take a short break by walking up and down the hall, then return to work refreshed.

Some adults with ADHD have difficulty sitting still for long periods of time and if forced to do so may unconsciously do things like fidgeting that annoy their coworkers. Individuals for whom this is true should first consider what type of a job would be a good fit for them. Not all jobs are in offices, and many careers (teaching, health care, sales, etc.) allow the worker to move around during a normal work day. If an office job is otherwise a good match, the individual can help themselves by being aware of their tendency and by scheduling periodic breaks into their day, during which time they get up and walk around (which can be disguised as getting water, using the restroom, etc., if necessary).

People with ADHD often have trouble with remembering things, particularly information provided verbally and informally. They can help themselves by taking detailed notes of meetings, using a planner that indicates when different projects are due, and setting up automatic reminders through an app that tells them what deadlines are coming up. They can also form the habit of clarifying anything that sounds like an assignment or a deadline at the time it is spoken, and then putting it in writing. Often coworkers and supervisors appreciate someone who is willing to take this additional step, and it can help a team to work together efficiently and harmoniously.

Many adults with ADHD struggle with time management and executive functions, and the use of planners and electronic aids can help with both issues. The specific system used is less important than the fact that the individual has committed to using it consistently and does so. A basic approach to long-term goals is to break them down into smaller goals with specific deadlines, and to set up reminders and task lists so it is clear which work takes the highest priority each day. Setting a timer to work for a specific length of time, followed by a break (the pomodoro system), works for many people in terms of organizing their work day. Some people also like to think in terms of large blocks of time, so certain hours of the day are devoted to specific projects. Some people also designate blocks of time during which they are not available for meetings or to respond to emails, so that they may be free to devote all their mental energies to a specific task.

Most jobs require a certain amount of interaction with coworkers, and this may pose challenges for people with ADHD. The first point is that people with ADHD need to be aware of how much personal interaction they want or can tolerate in their work day, and to choose jobs accordingly. It may also help to regard interpersonal communication as a skill that can be learned and practiced, rather than something that should come naturally. Observing how others in the workplace interact, and imitating them, can be helpful in learning the norms of a particular situation. Finally, counseling and coaching are available to help people learn and practice the conventions of conversation and other interpersonal interactions.

40. Can people with ADHD play sports?

People with ADHD both can and do play sports at all levels. While there is not a great deal of research into ADHD and participation in sports, some overviews have found that ADHD may occur at a higher rate in elite athletes than in the general population, possibly because some ADHD characteristics such as fast reaction time and the ability to shift attention quickly are beneficial in some sports. It may also be that some young people with ADHD do not function well in a classroom setting and find that sports provide a useful outlet for their energies and abilities. In addition, because success at sports is often valued highly by both peers and adults, excelling at a sport may provide a person with ADHD the kind of social approval and respect that they find difficult to achieve otherwise. Another possibility is that people with ADHD may respond particularly well to the strictly specified nature of a training regimen, with definite goals and highly organized scheduling.

There is some evidence that physical exercise can benefit children with ADHD by relieving some of their symptoms and improving executive function. Both sports and other forms of exercise (e.g., yoga, water aerobics) have been shown to have these benefits, so the choice may be based on what is available and what an individual prefers—some people like being part of a team and engaging in competition, while others like to exercise at their own pace and without the pressures that competition brings. Among the improvements found after engaging in exercise are improved attention, improved executive functioning, reduced anxiety and depression, reduced aggressive behavior, and improved motor functioning.

One specific consideration for athletes with ADHD is the status of any medications they may be prescribed. Stimulants are often used to treat ADHD, and some stimulants are prohibited by sport governing organizations because they are perceived to give the athlete taking them an unfair advantage. However, most organizations have therapeutic use exemptions for prescription medications, and if the appropriate steps are followed and the appropriate paperwork completed, the athlete can compete while taking their prescribed medications. Discontinuing medication in order to compete in a sport, without seeking medical advice, is as unwise as ceasing to take prescribed medication for any other reason. The specific rules to get a therapeutic use exemption vary from one organization to another, but often evidence of clinical diagnosis is typically required along with a statement from the prescribing physician specifying why the medications are necessary for the athlete. Some organizations may impose additional requirements, such as requiring routine monitoring and an annual reevaluation for specific medications. The purpose of these rules is not to punish or embarrass the athlete with ADHD but to ensure that competition conditions are fair for everyone.

The use of stimulants, even when prescribed, may raise concerns for the athlete or their parents. While it is true that stimulants may be abused, there is no evidence that treatment with prescribed stimulant medications is associated with any type of drug abuse, and medical guidelines specifically state that pharmacologic treatment should not be withheld on the grounds of potential abuse. Stimulants also raise the heart rate and blood pressure of the individuals taking them, but in most cases these effects are not sufficient to be a problem for an athlete. Of greater concern is the possible increased risk for sudden cardiac death (SCD) associated with taking stimulant medications. SCD is rare but extremely serious: as the name implies, it can cause death. Because SCD occurs in people with specific underlying conditions, including hypertrophic cardiomyopathy and Wolff-Parkinson-White syndrome, which under conditions of exertion can lead to uncontrolled ventricular arrhythmias, some countries require athletes to be screened by electrocardiogram for these underlying conditions before they can participate. However, this is not the case in the United States, due in part to the cost of widespread screening programs for conditions that are rare in the population, and in part due to inconsistent interpretation of electrocardiograms even among trained professionals.

Athletes taking prescribed stimulants are at higher than average risk of heat illness, which can cause death even in healthy young athletes. The increased risk is due to the way in which stimulants interfere with the body's thermoregulation system through changes in neurotransmitter activity. A person taking stimulants may be less aware of their rising temperature and fatigue, allowing them to continue to exercise longer and harder than they would without the stimulant, but also placing the athlete at increased risk of illness and death. Athletes taking stimulants therefore require extra monitoring and education about the risks and symptoms of heat illness to allow them to participate safely in their sport.

Some sports, such as American football, carry a high risk of concussion, so it is important for anyone with ADHD who participates in one of these sports, as well as their coaches and trainers, to be aware of how ADHD can interact with concussion protocols. The issue is not that people with ADHD are at greater risk for concussion but that the condition may interfere with evaluating the athlete before (baseline testing) and after a concussion, since ADHD can interfere with mental process such as memory, processing speed, and attention. There is some evidence that people with ADHD may recover more slowly from concussion than people without ADHD, although they do recover and there is no evidence that a concussion worsens ADHD symptoms or that taking prescribed stimulants interferes with recovery.

Participation in recreational or school sports in childhood is common among people both with and without ADHD, although there are some indications that people with ADHD may participate in recreational and school sports at a higher rate than those without ADHD. As with elite sports, there may be many reasons for this discrepancy, but it does establish that ADHD is no reason to forego participating in sport. People with ADHD may have an advantage in some sports due to fast reaction times and the ability to hyperfocus and may respond well to the more personal environment of a coached sport rather than a classroom. Sport also fosters different ways of interacting with both peers and adults, as compared to a classroom, and individuals who do well in sport can enjoy admiration and positive reinforcement that they may not have experienced in other settings.

A final piece of evidence that ADHD does not preclude participation in sport is the number of high-achieving athletes who have chosen to disclose that they have ADHD. Simone Biles, a multiple gold-medal winner in gymnastics at the Olympic and World level, spoke openly about taking Ritalin for her ADHD after a Russian computer hack revealed her private medical information. Swimmer Michael Phelps, who has won more Olympic medals than any other athlete, was diagnosed with ADHD as a child and has said that competing in sports helped him deal with the condition. Terry Bradshaw, an NFL quarterback who won four Super Bowls with the Pittsburgh Steelers and then enjoyed a successful career as a broadcaster, was diagnosed with ADHD in adulthood and discusses in his autobiography how being diagnosed earlier might have helped him do better in school as a child. Cammi Granato, a gold medalist in women's ice hockey for the United States, was also diagnosed with ADHD as an adult, and has stated that the condition is an essential part of who she is. Nicola Adams, a British boxer who won multiple gold medals in the Olympics before becoming a successful professional fighter, was diagnosed with ADHD as a teenager and says she thinks it has helped her succeed at her sport. Kevin Garnett, a basketball star inducted into the NBA Hall of Fame, was diagnosed late in his career, and has said that receiving the diagnosis helped him understand his early difficulties in focusing and learning to read.

41. I want to join the military—is that possible if I have ADHD?

American military policy concerning individuals with ADHD over the years has changed, so the answer to this question could also change. As of 2024, people with ADHD can serve in the military unless they have obvious symptoms or have taken medication for ADHD in the past year. In other words, the specifics of each individual case matter, and the best source of up-to-date information is the branch of the military in which the individual wants to enroll.

The military has recruiting offices in many locations around the United States, and often recruiters have a presence at events such as fairs, where they set up a table or booth and are available to speak with potential recruits. Information about recruitment is also available through the internet, and recruiters sometimes visit schools as well. A new recruit must meet two sets of criteria to be eligible for service: skills and aptitudes, and physical standards. Both are normally evaluated at a Military Entrance and Processing Station, although the skills and aptitudes exam may also be taken at satellite locations.

Skills and aptitudes for military service are evaluated through a written exam, the Armed Services Vocational Aptitude Battery (ASVAB), which is timed and for which no accommodations are allowed. The ASVAB exists in both computerized and pencil-and-paper forms, and scores achieved are comparable whichever means of administration was used. The computerized ASVAB is adaptive, meaning the computer selects questions for each applicant depending on whether previous questions were answered correctly or incorrectly, so different individuals may be asked different questions. The paper-and-pencil ASVAB is in fixed form; that is, everyone takes the same test. Each section or battery in the ASVAB has a time limit, and there is also a time limit for the total exam (198 minutes for the computerized version, 149 minutes for the paper-and-pencil version).

Ten content areas cover four domains (verbal, math, science and technical, and spatial) in the ASVAB, and each area is evaluated by a separate test within the battery. The areas are general science, arithmetic reasoning, work knowledge, paragraph comprehension, mathematics knowledge, electronics information, auto information, shop information, mechanical comprehension, and assembling objects. It is possible for applicants to prepare for the ASVAB, using information found online or in test preparation books available at bookstores, public libraries, and school libraries.

Enlistees must also pass a physical exam conducted by a military physician, who will also take a complete medical and psychiatric history of each applicant. The physical standards for enlistment are stated in a Department of Defense Directive (the most recent is DoD Instruction 6130.03, issued in 2018), which includes a list of conditions which disqualify an individual from military service. ADHD is listed in section 6.28 (Learning, Psychiatric, and Behavioral Disorders), which states that it is a disqualifying condition if any of four conditions are met: the individual has been recommended or prescribed an IEP (Individualized Education Program) after age 14, has a history of comorbid mental disorders, has been prescribed medication in the previous 24 months, or has documentation of adverse academic, occupational, or work performance. If none of those conditions apply, an individual with ADHD may be eligible to enlist, if they meet all other relevant standards. It is a crime to withhold or falsify information during the enlistment process, so it is best to be open and accurate when providing one's medical history. It is also true that individual branches of the military (e.g., the Army or the Navy) may grant waivers to individuals who don't meet the general military standards, although this is handled on an individual basis and is not guaranteed in any particular case.

Independent of meeting the qualifications to enlist, people with ADHD may want to consider whether they would thrive in a military environment, which can be quite different from other working and living environments. Answering this question requires research into how military training is conducted as well as what life is like when serving in the military, and speaking with people currently serving can provide valuable information. It's worth bearing in mind that the job of military recruiters is to recruit enlistees, and they have quotas to meet, so they may provide a more pleasant picture of military life than the recruit will actually experience. For this reason, speaking with people currently serving who are not recruiters can be a particularly valuable way to gain unbiased information.

Sometimes people with ADHD receive a diagnosis after they have enlisted, which may be due to either their concealing a previous diagnosis or simply never having been evaluated in civilian life. Given that the United States does not guarantee access to health care, and even insured people may find it difficult to access appropriate mental health and psychiatric care, such an outcome is not surprising. Researchers David Sayers, Zheng Hu, and Leslie L. Clark studied a sample of enlistees with ADHD to see how they fared as compared to enlistees without ADHD. The enlistees in this sample enlisted in 2014, during which time ADHD was a disqualifying condition if certain criteria were met, including long-term use of ADHD medication after age 14. Since all members of the study sample successfully enlisted, they passed the ASVAB, did not meet any of the disqualifying criteria (or did not fully disclose their condition), and did not display disqualifying symptoms during the military physical exam. They were matched on age, gender, and date of accession with active military members without an ADHD diagnosis, and military records for both groups were examined through 2018 or until they left the military.

Sayers and colleagues studied 996 service members who enlisted in 2014 and were identified as having ADHD after that point. About one-third of the groups was prescribed ADHD medication; the treated groups were more likely to be female, age 20 or older, members of racial or ethnic minority groups, junior officers, and to be enlisted in the Army. After eliminating anyone who left the military within 6 months of enlistment, the researchers had a study sample of 616 individuals, of whom 331 were treated with medication; the non-ADHD group decreased to 911 after removing individuals who left the military within 6 months of enlistment. Attrition for service members with ADHD was much higher in the first 6 months, as compared to service members without ADHD, and the ADHD group who received treatment had the highest attrition rates, possibly because their symptoms were the most severe. The group receiving treatment for ADHD also had significantly higher rates of mental health disorders, with the greatest difference observed for anxiety disorders, while the group with untreated ADHD did not have a significantly different rate of mental health disorders as compared to those without ADHD.

One reality of military life is the possibility of receiving assignments that require the individual to move, possibly to another state or country. While there are some differences between the different branches of the military, in general an enlisted person is assigned a permanent duty station, which could be in the United States or overseas. Individuals may also be assigned to serve in a different location for a short period of time (temporary duty assignment) or for a permanent change of station. While expenses to move the enlisted individual and their family are covered by the military, and there are some commonalities among military bases no matter where they are located, moving can be stressful for people with ADHD.

The possibility of frequent moves, and of temporary separation of household members, should be considered for parents serving in the military who have a child or other household member who has ADHD. Educational and medical services will be available wherever the enlisted member is transferred, but children with ADHD may find it particularly stressful to adapt to a new school, a new doctor, and so on. Military parents can help ease the transition for their child with ADHD by preparing them mentally for the move, following a routine, helping the child stay in touch with old friends and meet new ones, being proactive about contacting the child's new school and new physician, and sharing educational and medical records as appropriate. If a child has an IEP in their current school, their new school must provide comparable services, although the new school may develop a new IEP if they deem it necessary after conducting their own evaluation of the child.

42. What are some of the common social problems for people with ADHD?

People with ADHD often experience problems with social functioning, including difficulties in forming appropriate relationships with peers and authority figures, and these difficulties are experienced by adults as well as children. Being unable to function socially in ways that are expected and considered normal in a society can have wide-ranging impacts on an individual, from interfering with success at school or at work to loneliness and constant frustration at the inability to do something which is an expected part of everyday human life and appears to be simple and obvious for most people.

Because most research on ADHD has been conducted on children and adolescents, we know much more about the kinds of social issues they experience, as well as what kind of interventions may prove most useful for them. For adults, there is less research, but with increasing awareness that ADHD can be a lifetime condition, more researchers are starting to turn their attention to adults with ADHD and there is more interest in developing interventions that are effective for adults with ADHD.

Successful social interactions require the ability to understand and follow conventions which most people learn unconsciously as they mature. Because these conventions seem natural to those who have learned them, any departure from the conventions may be misinterpreted. In this way, impulsive behavior may be seen as rudeness, failure to respond to an invitation as unfriendliness, and so on. For reasons we don't entirely understand, some people with ADHD seem to not learn social conventions or be unable to follow them, resulting in misunderstandings that can make the person with ADHD a social outcast. Even if some of the conventions seem arbitrary or unfair, it's important to learn how to function within them in order to have normal social relationships with people. Fortunately, it's possible to learn how to interact in conventional social ways, even if it seems unnatural or arbitrary, and the rewards of doing so make the effort worthwhile. Some people with ADHD can learn these skills deliberately on their own, or with informal assistance from friends and family, while others may choose to take social skills training with a psychologist or other trained professional.

For a person with ADHD, difficulties in social interaction often begin in childhood peer interactions. Children with inattentive symptoms may miss social cues, be easily distracted, or have difficulty in listening to others. While this behavior may be unintentional on the part of the child with ADHD, to other children it may seem like rudeness or self-centeredness. As a result, the child with ADHD may find themselves without friends and the target of teasing and bullying. Hyperactive symptoms associated with ADHD can result in breaches of social convention such as excessive talking or the inability to take turns in conversation, behaviors which may be unintentional but do not make the child a desirable conversation partner. Impulsive behavior, ranging from aggression to clownish behavior at inappropriate times, as well as social breaches such as failing to respect other people's personal space are likely to be met with disapproval from authority figures as well as peers.

Unfortunately, when such patterns are established, they may prove resistant to change. As a result, a child with ADHD may go through childhood without forming any close peer relationships. Isolation can lead to frustration and more acting out, as well as becoming afraid to initiate social interactions since the child has learned they are likely to be rejected. A child who can't form good peer relationships misses out on the chance to further develop their social skills through interactions and to develop a sense of belonging and acceptance. Such a child may also be labeled as difficult and uncooperative by their teachers, a label that may become a self-fulfilling prophecy. Lack of social skills can also impair academic progress, particularly in schools where group or team projects are an important part of the curriculum, while difficulties in conversation may make it difficult for a child to know how to appropriately ask for help when they need it.

Social difficulties do not simply disappear with age for people with ADHD, although adults may be more able to control some tendencies, such as hyperactivity, that make social interactions difficult. On the other hand, the tolerance that may be extended to children due to their lack of maturity is unlikely to apply to adults, and so an adult who displays behaviors like interrupting or failing to listen when others are speaking is even more likely to be labeled as rude and self-centered. Such a person may find that others don't want to be friends with them or to have them a member of their work group. Since ADHD is an invisible disability, it's understandable that people will make such judgments, and the burden is not inappropriately placed on the person with ADHD to learn how to interact in a conventional manner.

Medication and general counseling may help people with ADHD control their symptoms, but people experiencing difficulties in social interactions may also seek out specialized training in social skills. Some schools offer training in social skills, and psychologists and other trained professionals may also offer it in private practice. Such training usually involves setting specific goals based on the needs of the client and their maturity level, such as learning to listen and engage in conversation, learning how to enter new group situations, or learning positive ways to cope with boredom or frustration. The goal is to help the person with ADHD learn and practice social conventions so they can interact in an expected manner with others. Social skills sessions can take a variety of forms, depending on the client's needs, the therapist's training, and the age of the client, but may include role-playing, coaching, observing and explaining short videos of appropriate behavior, and practicing the techniques learned in a safe environment before trying them in the real world. If the client is a child, the parent may also receive training in how to help their child learn and practice social behaviors.

43. How can ADHD impact romantic relationships?

Most adults experience the desire to have romantic and/or sexual relationships with other people, and many want to have a long-term partner, whether within a marriage or outside of it. People with ADHD have similar desires, but due to symptoms of their condition often experience difficulties in social interaction that make dating and successful engaging in romantic or sexual relationships difficult.

In the United States, romantic partnerships, including marriage, are generally considered to be based on the mutual agreement of the people involved. It means that both members of a relationship must actively choose to be in it, and either one can choose to end it. Different people want different things out of a relationship, but many people want a partner who is committed to the relationship, who makes the effort to understand the other member of the relationship, and takes their needs and desires into account. Maintaining a good intimate relationship is not easy and requires both maturity and a willingness to communicate with the partner. It also often gets better with practice, so people often say that their relationship deepens as they and their partner learn how to live with each other.

For people with ADHD, trouble with romantic relationship often begins in the teenage years, as they pass through puberty. This is the time which (in most communities) is considered appropriate to begin to express feelings of love or affection and to begin dating, although marriage and sexual relationships may still be some years in the future. It's a time when many people learn about their own desires and decide what they want in a partner, and also when they gain experience in expressing their feelings and listening to and understanding the feelings of those they are attracted to. It's also a time when many young people talk to their peers about who they like and how they feel about them, and peer support as well as parental guidance helps them learn appropriate ways to express and respond to romantic feelings. Schools and institutions such as churches often arrange social events, such as dances, to provide a safe and chaperoned place for young people to explore and express their romantic feelings.

People with ADHD sometimes find themselves excluded from the dating scene in adolescence due to their difficulties with communication and tendency to not notice or respond appropriately to social cues. If they don't gain the social experiences their peers do at this age, they may well enter adulthood without having had the chance to develop a mature understanding of their own desires or to practice socially appropriate ways of expressing and receiving expressions of desire. The result may be an adult who knows less about appropriate behavior in the context of dating and romance than a typical teenager, and this lack of knowledge and experience is likely to continue to result in frustration and lack of success in finding partners.

In some ways the difficulties that many people with ADHD have with social interactions are magnified in romantic relationships, where even greater attentiveness to social norms and to subtle social cures is expected. To look at matters from the point of view of a potential romantic partner who does not have ADHD, it's easy to see why they might find dating or being in a relationship with a person with ADHD exasperating, no matter how sympathetic or well informed they are about the condition. They're not running a social charity but seeking to be in a rewarding relationship, and it's perfectly reasonable to want to be with someone whose company they enjoy and who can express their feelings and desire to be in the relationship. ADHD characteristics like forgetting about dates, drifting off mentally in the midst of a conversation, shifting conversation topics abruptly, or dressing inappropriately for social situations are likely to be interpreted as signs of a lack of interest in the relationship or as simple rudeness. People with ADHD sometimes have sensory difficulties as well, and since romantic relationships usually involve touching, this may be an obstacle to dating and forming romantic relationships as well.

In a relationship in which one person has ADHD and the other does not, there are some things the person who does not have ADHD can do to help the relationship. One is to understand that the partner's behavior may well not be meant as a personal insult, and the partner may in fact be unaware that what they are doing is hurtful. That does not suggest that the partner need ignore or accept the behavior but that they may need to inform the person with ADHD what they are doing and why it is hurtful. The partner can also inform themselves about ADHD and how it can affect behavior. They can also join a support group for partners of people with ADHD if one is available in their area (or join an online community with that focus). Looking for solutions (e.g., using a shared planner for scheduling, keeping a list of what chores each person will be responsible for and how often they will be done) is more productive than responding with anger or hurt to misunderstanding. Both parties may need to work on communication (again, this is common for many couples, even if ADHD is not involved) and commit to making the relationship work. No one is obliged to stay in a bad relationship, and both parties need to be aware of their limits. The partner can also attend counseling or coaching to help them understand the person with ADHD and interact more successfully with them.

If a person with ADHD has symptoms that make socializing difficult, they may want to mention their condition to a potential partner fairly early in the relationship and explain how it affects their behavior and the way they experience the world. This should not be framed as making excuses for apparent bad behavior, but as an honest attempt to communicate with the partner about themselves. It is also incumbent on a person with ADHD to seek appropriate care, do the best they can to control symptoms that could be interpreted as antisocial or rude, and learn and practice the conventions of interacting with others in their society. Counseling and coaching may be useful to help the person with ADHD succeed in social and romantic relationships, and a couple in which one or both partners have ADHD may also find they benefit from marriage or couples counseling with a therapist knowledgeable about ADHD.

Some of the techniques recommended for organization in a workplace or educational context can help a person with ADHD succeed in forming and maintaining relationships. For instance, one can use a planner to record upcoming social events, set electronic reminders, and use a timer or set an alarm to ensure promptness. Planning aspects of dating in advance, such as what to wear, can be helpful in adhering to social conventions. Developing an understanding of what kinds of social situations cause distress (e.g., noisy parties, crowds at sporting events) is also helpful, and planning can help the person with ADHD choose social situations in which they do feel comfortable. Awareness of one's specific needs, and planning socially acceptable ways to meet them, is also useful. For instance, a person who knows they can't sit still for hours at a time needs to plan activities that allow them to move around at regular intervals. While dealing with some of these issues may seem like a lot of work, it's worth doing if you want to have a successful and lasting romantic relationship. In a way, people with ADHD are just dealing with a more extreme versions of the kind of self-knowledge, disclosure, and negotiation that every couple must deal with, and being honest with yourself and any potential partners about what you like and don't like, and what you can and can't do, is a good way to improve the chances of having a successful and lasting relationship.

44. What does it mean to self-medicate, and why might it be harmful?

When a person self-medicates, it means they are using a substance, such as alcohol, to deal with symptoms or other problems that are not effectively being treated. The self-medication is a symptom of an underlying problem, such as ADHD, and a two-pronged approach may be necessary: treat the underlying condition, and also help the person deal with issues caused by the self-medication.

Some of the substances used for self-medication are also used without problems by many adults, so identifying self-medication is usually a matter of why the person is using a substance and how it is affecting their lives. Self-medication is often identified after it has begun to cause problems for the person: for instance, a person may drink to hide symptoms of social anxiety, but in the process finds they act inappropriately while drunk and find themselves even more isolated than before. To take another example, a person who drinks to feel less nervous at a party may drive home in an inebriated condition, potentially causing an accident or being arrested for driving under the influence. The substance used to self-medicate does not need to be illegal: alcohol, caffeine, and nicotine (a substance found in tobacco products such as cigarettes and chewing tobacco), which are legal in at least some circumstances, can be used to self-medicate. Prescription drugs not prescribed to the person taking them can also be used to self-medicate. There's some evidence that there may be genetic reasons why some people are more likely than others to abuse substances, and condemning the individual user is not an effective approach to dealing with the problem. Instead, it is generally more effective to treat any underlying conditions, such as ADHD, that may be causing the person to self-medicate, and to refer them to medical or psychological counseling if necessary.

Self-medication is a concern for people with ADHD for several reasons. The first is that it may prevent the person from seeking medical treatment which might be more effective and less harmful. In countries like the United States, which doesn't have a system of National Health, this is a particular issue because not everyone has health insurance that allows them to see a physician or get prescriptions fill. A second problem is that self-medication may be ineffective and mask rather than solve the underlying problem. For instance, some people have anxiety about being in situations in which they're expected to interact socially with others and may drink alcohol to feel less anxious. This approach may help with the symptoms of anxiety and nervousness, but doesn't address the underlying problem, which is the person needs to learn how to interact socially. It may actually make the underlying problem worse, because the person may act inappropriately while intoxicated or get labeled as a drunk, making other people even less interested in socializing with them.

A third problem is that the substance used to self-medicate may be harmful. For instance, excessive drinking can have a number of bad health outcomes, while using alcohol as way to control anxiety can lead to a dependency which may be difficult to treat. Similarly, a person who smokes to help them concentrate may find themselves addicted to the nicotine in tobacco, and tobacco use is associated with a higher risk for a number of diseases. A fourth problem is that self-medication may get the person into trouble with the law. Some substances used to self-medicate are illegal (e.g., marijuana in some states, alcohol for people younger than 21), and some are illegal under certain circumstances (e.g., driving while intoxicated).

Some of the substances used to self-medicate are not necessarily harmful but can be so if used to excess. For example, many adults consume caffeine daily, often in the form of coffee or tea, without experiencing any side effects. There's some evidence that people with ADHD may on average consume more caffeine than people without ADHD, and some people with ADHD believe consuming caffeine helps them to concentrate (the evidence is mixed on this question). Consuming caffeine per se is not a problem for most adults, unless a person has a specific health risk, religious prohibition, and so on. However, consuming too much caffeine can lead to a variety of problems, including disturbed sleep patterns, elevated blood pressure, and a rapid heart rate. People can develop a tolerance for caffeine so that over time they need to take more of it; for example, drink more coffee, to get the same effect. It is also possible to overdose on caffeine, which may produce symptoms like vomiting, rapid or irregular heartbeat, and hallucinations. Because the body adapts to caffeine consumption, people who stop consuming caffeine suddenly may also develop withdrawal symptoms such as headaches and problems with concentration, although these usually subside over a few days.

For young people, caffeine use is more of a concern, particularly since many common foods and beverages, as well as some over-the-counter medications, include caffeine. The American Academy of Child and Adolescent Psychiatry advises that children under 12 not consume caffeine at all, and that children aged 12–18 consume no more than 100 milligrams of caffeine daily. Often young people consume caffeine through sodas, energy drinks, and energy shots, whose caffeine content can vary widely, so it is necessary to read the label to see how much caffeine any given size and brand contains. Sweetened coffee and tea drinks are also popular with some young people, and some of these drinks contain over 200 mg of caffeine in a single serving, which is twice what is recommended for people age 18 and younger. Independent of the amount of caffeine contained in a beverage, users should observe their own reactions and adjust their behavior accordingly. For instance, if a 20-ounce brewed coffee makes you feel shaky, try ordering a smaller drink next time or split the larger drink with a friend. Many popular coffee and tea drinks are also available in decaffeinated form another possibility for people sensitive to caffeine.

People with ADHD sometimes use alcohol to self-medicate symptoms such as restlessness, anxiety, and impulsivity, or to make themselves forget about problems that may be related to their ADHD, such as workplace or academic failure. While many adults can drink a moderate amount of alcohol without problems, masking symptoms through alcohol use rather than dealing with the underlying condition by seeking appropriate treatment for ADHD is not a good idea. Alcohol use sometimes increases ADHD symptoms, including inattentiveness and impulsivity, and can interact with some medications. Drinking alcohol can reduce people's inhibitions, and they may do something while under the influence that they would not have if sober. Alcohol consumption also reduces coordination and reduces alertness, and may cause distortions in vision and hearing, all of which explain why driving or operating heavy machinery while drunk is generally prohibited. Excessive alcohol use can lead to blackouts, memory lapses, or even death, and prolonged alcohol abuse is associated with a number of bad outcomes including liver disease, increased risk for some cancers, and digestive issues. If alcohol is causing a person problems, medical and/or psychological health should be sought, because there are many different treatment programs that can help a person reduce or eliminate alcohol use.

People with ADHD may also use nicotine, which is found in tobacco products such as cigarettes, cigars, and chewing tobacco, to self-medicate. Tobacco use increases the risk for many serious diseases and conditions, including heart attack, stroke, vascular disease, and lung cancer, and exposure to second-hand smoke (i.e., inhaling the smoke produced by someone else who is smoking) is also associated with increased health risks, particularly for children, including SIDS (sudden infant death syndrome), middle ear disease, acute respiratory infections, and asthma. For these reasons, people who smoke are often counseled to stop, although this can be difficult because nicotine is addictive and those who stop smoking may experience withdrawal symptoms. A medical professional or counselor can help a smoker through the process of quitting, and there are many different programs available to help people stop smoking. Some people also find that either prescription or over-the-counter medications (e.g., nicotine replacement patches or gum) may help them through the process. Interestingly, some research has found that smokers with ADHD who received effective ADHD medication smoked less and improved their ability to concentrate, so seeking appropriate treatment for the underlying condition of ADHD may also help smokers with ADHD cut back on their tobacco consumption or quit entirely.

45. There are people in my life that don't believe ADHD is real. How can I help them understand that it is a legitimate condition and how it affects me?

When people think of diseases or disorders, their first thoughts are likely to be of well-known medical diseases like strep throat or chicken pox, which can be identified through lab tests and can be cured through specific treatments. Those kinds of diseases feel very concrete and real, and few people would try to argue to someone with a throat infection that it's all in their head. Most people experience multiple medical diseases during their lives and thus are less inclined to dismiss their existence. However, mental conditions and disorders such as ADHD may be less familiar to many people, and they may have less understanding of how a condition like ADHD can affect someone's functioning. The complications involved with diagnosing and treating ADHD can also cause people to question if it is real—although ADHD may be caused by physical differences in people's brains, there's no simple lab test to make a diagnosis. Another issue is that the symptoms of mental conditions or disorders, including ADHD, are not always distinct to the condition but occur in many people, with the severity and frequency of the symptoms being important criteria in making a diagnosis.

Some people simply have a bias against the existence of mental disorders, and others may believe that such a diagnosis did not exist in their childhood—it is not valid. If a person doesn't believe that ADHD is real, they may ascribe some of the behaviors caused by it to character flaws or a lack of discipline and believe that the person affected should simply "snap out of it" and stop behaving badly. Another reason they may be suspicious of the reality of ADHD is that there have been highly publicized cases where someone successfully pretended to have ADHD in order to win advantages for themselves, and as a result they doubt that anyone's ADHD is real. None of these criticisms are fair, of course, but they certainly exist, and can be particularly hurtful if the person holding the uninformed opinion is a friend or family member. The ubiquity of the internet and various forms of social media today make it easy to spread false information about ADHD, which may seem very convincing if the person has no context for judging it, and for people who believe that ADHD is not real to reinforce each other's opinions in a sort of echo chamber. Some people seem to believe that repeating confrontational talking points ("Giving your child Ritalin is child abuse!") makes them seem smart or that refusing to consider other opinions or information is a sign of mental discipline. If you encounter such a person, it may not be worth your while to try to reason with them.

Clearly, there's a lot of work to do regarding teaching people about mental conditions and disorders, but it's not reasonable to expect people with ADHD to take on that task single-handedly. For young children, this task may be best handled by a parent or other adult, although they can also give the child a brief explanation to use with their friends or anyone else they need to inform. Mature teenagers and adults can take on the task of educating others if they choose to do so, but it must be their own choice and not something that is simply expected of them because they have the condition. After all, we don't demand that a person with a cancer also assume the burden of explaining it to others, although some may elect to do so. If you decide to engage in discussion, it's wise to consider what outcome you want from it and whether that is likely to be achieved. While some people are open to listening to evidence and changing their minds, some are not, and sometimes it's better to agree to disagree than to get in an argument. A medical professional or counselor may be able to help the person with ADHD formulate an explanation appropriate to their maturity level, and there are many factsheets and similar information written for nonprofessionals available online that may help in crafting an answer or an explanation about what ADHD is.

If you have decided to take on the task of explaining ADHD to someone who doesn't believe in it, and determined that there's a good chance the outcome of the conversation will be positive, one good point to begin with is that numerous scientific and medical groups, including the National Institutes of Health, the Centers for Disease Control and Prevention, the American Medical Association, and the American Psychiatric Association, all agree that ADHD is a valid condition that can be helped with treatment. International health organizations such as the World Health Organization also agree that ADHD is both real and treatable. You could also point out that there are standard procedures for diagnosing ADHD, as outlined in the *DSM* (the *Diagnostic and Statistical Manual of the American Psychiatric Association*), and that not everyone who is evaluated for ADHD is diagnosed as having it. The fact that some people have faked a diagnosis or been able to influence a clinician to give them a diagnosis that was not warranted should not be used to discredit the many people with ADHD who have engaged in no such deception.

Sometimes people question the existence of ADHD because it was unknown when they were young or at least it wasn't as well-known as it is today. They may also be suspicious after reading reports about how diagnosis with ADHD has become more common in recent years, asking how such a disorder could suddenly appear or become common in a population where it was rare or unknown a few generations earlier. The best approach in this case may be to focus on explaining how the process of medical and psychiatric diagnosis is not constant like the laws of mathematics but is always changing in response to new information. The same could be said of many medical procedures: for instance organ transplants were once the stuff of science fiction, then were a groundbreaking and rare procedure in the 1950s, and today are a commonplace life-saving procedure. The changes are due to a combination of factors, including increased scientific understanding, improvements in drug therapies, and a national system for allocating organs. In the case of ADHD, diagnostic criteria have been modified as the medical community learned more about the condition and as original assumptions (such that it being primarily a condition that occurred in young boys) have been proven false. As people have learned more about ADHD, and as better treatments became available, more have chosen to have themselves evaluated for it, resulting in a diagnosis when a few decades prior they wouldn't have even made the appointment for evaluation.

Some people are also suspicious of an ADHD diagnosis because the symptoms of ADHD are not unique but may also be considered part of the spectrum of normal behavior. This is true but is not unique to ADHD: for instance, diagnosis with the autoimmune disorder is based on the degree of difference from the norm in certain hormones, and there is no absolute line separating the ill from the well. In the case of ADHD, the process of diagnosis usually involves multiple sources of information, including a medical history, direct observation of behavior, and psychological testing. It might also be useful to mention the improvements in symptoms, and more generally in life outcomes, experienced by people with ADHD when their condition is diagnosed and treated appropriately, and the fact that a person who is treated appropriately for ADHD is generally also easier for others to be around, whether they are a child in school, an adult in a job, or a member of a family at any age.

It is never required for a person to share personal details of their life in order to justify their existence. However, if you feel comfortable and secure doing so, you may choose to share what it has been like for you to have ADHD and how being diagnosed and treated has made things better for you. This is most advisable for an adolescent or adult rather than a child, because it can feel like an invasion of privacy, and can be particularly difficult if the person you are speaking to continues to question your own experience of life and insist that you are mistaken or misled about your own reality. No one should ever be put in that position (it's a form of gaslighting and can lead a person to doubt the evidence of their own senses), and if a person continues to deny that ADHD exists, that may be a good indication that it's time to end the discussion. The same advice applies if the other person becomes insulting or abusive—it's too bad they don't want to learn, but it's not necessarily your job to teach them.

46. Where can I find support to help me deal with ADHD?

One good thing about having ADHD today is that there are far more resources and support available than in the past. There are really two aspects to finding support: one is finding professional help from physician, psychologist, or other medical professional trained in evaluating and treating people with ADHD. Professional legal help may also be required, for instance, to advocate for a student with ADHD to receive the accommodations and support to which they are entitled. The second is finding self-help resources, some of which may have been created by professionals but are written in terms a layman can understand,

and others of which are created by people with ADHD who want to share their experiences to help others. While there's no substitute for competent professional evaluation and treatment, many people find that "own voices" stories (those written by people who have the characteristic featured, in this case someone with ADHD writing about what it's like to have ADHD) are also useful in understanding themselves and learning ways to navigate through the world.

To find professional help, the best starting point may be the family physician or school counselor, who may be able to recommend a physician or psychologist in the area. A local university may also be a source of good information, particularly if the university has a medical school or offers a Ph.D. program in education, counseling, or psychology. Several ADHD organizations have online directories that allow searching for professionals who have experience with ADHD, including CHADD (Children and Adults with Attention Deficit/ Hyperactivity Disorder, which hosts the National Resource Center for ADHD), the Council of Parent Attorneys and Advocates, and the Special Needs Alliance, all of whose websites are listed in the Directory of Resources. Several websites created by entitles within the federal government, including the Department of Education and the Department of Labor, are also designed to help people understand their rights and to access the benefits to which they are entitled. These websites are also listed in the Directory of Resources. A simple internet search may also help locate professional resources, although of course judgment is required when evaluating anything found through an internet search, because there's a lot of misinformation and scams out there and the results produced by a search engine (e.g., Google) are not curated in the way information from a reliable website will be.

Several professional organizations also maintain websites or web pages with information about ADHD written for nonprofessionals. The type of resources one may find on such websites is wide-ranging and may include simple explanations of ADHD, typical difficulties experienced by people with ADHD, treatments available, fact sheets and statistical data about ADHD, and advice on coping with ADHD. Often this information is available in different formats, including as print, videos, and sound recordings. Sometimes it is available in different languages as well. Some websites organize information according to the intended audience—for children with ADHD, parents of children with ADHD, adolescents with ADHD, adults with ADHD, and so on—with the information presented in each section tailored for that group. Examples of professional organizations who maintain websites with information written for laypersons include CHADD, the American Academy of Pediatrics, the American Academy for Child and Adolescent Psychiatry, the American Psychological Association, and the Centers for Disease Control and Prevention, whose websites are listed in the Directory of Resources.

Many books have been written by people with ADHD, or by parents or other family members of someone with ADHD, with the purpose of sharing their experiences and helping others to understand this condition. While the advice contained in these books is not necessarily professionally vetted, they can still be useful in terms of helping people with ADHD recognize themselves in someone else's story and learning how that person found ways to succeed and find their own voice. A few books of this type are listed in the Directory of Resources, and many more can be found at public libraries or through an internet search. People with ADHD also have written many articles available through online publications like *ADDitude* (website listed in the Directory of Resources). While not a substitute for professional advice, publications such as *Additude* may help people with ADHD see how other people with the condition experience life and learn the ways they have found to help them deal with a world in which many people don't understand ADHD.

Some organizations also maintain online forums for people with ADHD and others who want to share their experiences with the condition. These forums are another way to access "own voices" narratives about ADHD, and as such can be very useful in helping people with ADHD understand themselves and their condition, as well as finding useful tips about coping in the world. Since the posts on these forums typically don't come from trained professionals, any advice offered should be evaluated with that in mind, but they can prove very useful in helping people with ADHD find community with others that share their condition.

The largest forum for ADHD is maintained on the Reddit website, which also includes many more specific forums for different classes of people, including women with ADHD, partners of people with ADHD, parents of children with ADHD, and college students with ADHD, and to discuss different ADHD medications. A few of these forums are private, meaning it is necessary to apply to join in order to post and see posts, but others are available to anyone with access to a computer and a web browser. Of course, that means you need to take extra care in considering anything posted on the public forums, because they sometimes attract people who are dishonest or who are out to cause trouble rather than contributing productively to a conversation. Several other organizations offering online forums are listed in the Directory of Resources, and more can be located through an internet search, but the caveats about anything found through an internet search apply to forums as well: the burden is on the reader to evaluate whatever they find there, and they are not a substitute for professional help.

47. Are there advantages to having ADHD?

Often ADHD is considered as a handicap or deficit in contrast to what is considered "normal" (not having ADHD). Another way to look at ADHD is to consider the advantages that may come from having it. Some people with ADHD describe it as a "superpower" that gives them an edge over other people and has helped them succeed. The fact that some people with ADHD have been outstandingly successful in their lives should offer encouragement to anyone who is struggling to adapt to a world that is not always ready to accept them. Of course, each person with ADHD is a unique individual with a specific combination of talents and personality traits, so it would be wrong to try to impose a template for ADHD success, but learning about traits common to ADHD and how they may connect to success in the world may be useful for anyone with ADHD, particularly when it comes to deciding on a career path.

There are many lists of famous people with ADHD on the internet, but they should be evaluated with the understanding that such lists can be based on speculation. However, many celebrities have chosen to speak publicly about having ADHD, and reading about their lives and the adaptations they made to their condition can be useful to other people with ADHD. Examples of celebrities with ADHD who have chosen to share information about their experiences with ADHD include Emma Watson (actor), Michelle Rodriguez (actor), Henry Winkler (actor), Jim Carrey (actor), Scott Kelly (astronaut), Simone Biles (athlete), Michael Phelps (athlete), Terry Bradshaw (actor and broadcaster), Will.i.am (musician), Britney Spears (musician and songwriter), Adam Levine (musician and actor), Justin Timberlake (musician and actor), Mel B (musician), Greta Gerwig (actor, writer, and director), James Carville (political consultant), Howie Mandel (comedian and actor), Channing Tatum (actor), Audra McDonald (musician and actor), Paul Orfalea (founder of Kinko's), Robin Black (author), Dav Pilkey (author), Sir Richard Branson (founder of the Virgin Group), David Neeleman (businessman, founder of JetBlue Airways), and Ingvar Kamprad (founder of Ikea). It's also worth remembering that many successful people with ADHD are not celebrities, so their stories are not widely publicized.

When choosing a course of study or a career path, it's important to consider one's strengths as well as weaknesses. Unfortunately, for people with ADHD the focus has often been on the latter, with emphasis on how differences from what is considered "normal" can limit a person's life choices and success. It's equally valid to focus on strengths and to consider what a person with ADHD is or can be really good at. This requires an honest inventory on the part of the individual, although career counselors who are well-informed about ADHD may also be helpful.

For instance, a person with hyperfocus may do exceptionally well in jobs such as scientific research or computer programming, which require extended concentration to work on exacting problems, and allow a high degree of independent work. A person who is full of energy and has difficulty being still may excel in sports or in other jobs that require a high level of physical activity. Someone who is spontaneous and creative may excel in fields commonly regarded as artistic, such as music, art, or writing, but may also do well in business or research where they can "think outside the box" to come up with solutions to problems that haven't occurred to anyone else. The self-knowledge required of people with ADHD, as well as the observational skills they may develop as a result of trying to fit in despite being different, can result in high levels of understanding and empathy for others, which may translate into success as a counselor, psychologist, or supervisor. The tendency to pay attention to things other people overlook, and to focus on details even if their importance is not obvious, can be useful in many careers, including academic and scientific research and criminal investigation.

Case Studies

Case 1. Sam Is Struggling in Third Grade and Doesn't Understand Why

Sam is an 8-year-old boy in third grade at a public elementary school in a middle-class suburb near a major city. Most parents in the community having professional jobs and are strong believers in the importance of their children's education, so the local school system is well funded through property taxes and many parents also take part in fundraising events to provide extras like class trips. The elementary school Sam attends is a bright and welcoming place with dedicated teachers who strive to treat each student as an individual. At the same time it is influenced by the demands of parents that the school system produce high achievers, particularly in academics. Students from the middle school and high school have done well in national competitions like the American Mathematical Olympiad and the FIRST Robotics Competition, and the high school graduation program lists where each student will be attending college.

Sam is a bright and friendly child who wants to please his parents, who are very invested in his education and future success. He attended a preschool based around creative play with other children from his neighborhood and had no difficulty fitting in with the other students. His first few years in elementary school were also unremarkable, and he impressed his teachers with his creativity and intelligence. Recently, however, Sam has begun to struggle in his classes, which have become more focused on structured academic lessons for the entire class, rather than letting students move between activities as they choose. He finds it difficult to stay seated at his desk and follow the lesson being taught and becomes bored and frustrated easily if he can't move around. He has also shown bursts of more disturbing behavior, including shouting and running around the classroom during lessons, although he is always remorseful once he has calmed down.

Sam's teacher was sufficiently alarmed by Sam's behavior, both the classroom disruptions and the fact that he is falling behind his classmates academically, to contact his parents, a university professor and a lawyer. They are concerned that Sam is having problems with school, which he used to love, although they are not clear about the source of the problem, since he comes home upset some days but doesn't want to talk about it. Although Sam is only in the third grade, they are concerned that he is not keeping up with the other students and wonder what could be behind what seems to them like an extreme change in attitude and behavior.

At the recommendation of his teacher, Sam's parents take him to a psychiatrist who is experienced in dealing with children having academic and behavioral issues. After a series of interviews, observations, and testing, the psychiatrist tells them that Sam is displaying characteristics of ADHD of the hyperactive-impulsive type, which is making it difficult for him to meet the expectations of his classroom teacher. The psychiatrist also tells them that the shift in emphasis at Sam's school, from self-motivated and informal activities to more formal academic instruction, may be adding to his difficulties, but is in no way an indication of a lack of intelligence or the ability to learn on Sam's part. He emphasizes that many people with ADHD go on to be high achievers in their chosen profession.

The psychiatrist tells Sam's parents that while many treatment options are available, he thinks they should begin with behavioral techniques. Sam's parents don't know much about ADHD and are rather shocked that their child could have what sounds like a serious mental illness. The psychiatrist refers them to a psychologist who specializes in helping families who have a young child with ADHD and assures them that they can learn ways to help Sam understand and control the symptoms of his condition, and that as he matures, he will be able to take on more of the responsibility of managing himself.

The psychologist, a Ph.D. in psychology who specializes in learning disabilities, begins by educating Sam's parents about ADHD. She refers to it as a "condition" rather than an "illness" or "disease" and encourages them to do likewise, particularly when speaking to Sam or his teacher. Like the psychiatrist, she emphasizes that ADHD need not be a barrier to success, but that because Sam's brain works differently from most people's, he will need extra help to organize himself. She introduces them to practical methods they can use to help structure his day, including creating a calendar with a daily schedule of activities and giving him clear instructions about any tasks he needs to complete. They also speak to his teacher, who is already knowledgeable about ADHD, and who agrees to help Sam learn to recognize his feelings and manage them. She agrees to give him extra support and creates a system in which, if he is feeling restless, he can ask for permission to move about the classroom as long as he does so in a way that does not disrupt the other students. Sam's parents and teacher schedule a series of meetings throughout the school year to discuss Sam's progress and collaborate to help him succeed.

Analysis

Sam's teacher did the right thing by being proactive and contacting his parents when he began to struggle in school, rather than letting him fall behind or become accustomed to playing the role of classroom disrupter. She suggested a specialist who could determine if there were mental or physical reasons underlying Sam's behavior and then suggest ways to move forward. Sam's parents, although highly educated, were not well-informed about ADHD but were willing to learn about it and to take an active role in helping their son learn to manage his condition. They realized that their son was not deliberately being bad but found it more difficult than most children his age to sit still and attend to a lesson. They also realized that his behavior was disrupting the classroom and could not simply be ignored or treated as something he would grow out of. So they worked with a specialist in learning disabilities to create a more structured environment for their son and to be more clear about their expectations. Sam's teacher also used behavior techniques to help Sam, including being more clear about instructions for each task and allowing him some freedom to accommodate his need to move about while setting boundaries so that he could do so in a socially acceptable manner. Both parents and teacher also agreed to meet regularly so they could discuss how Sam was faring, what was working and what wasn't, and make adjustments accordingly. While Sam's behavior did not change overnight, with patience and persistence he learned to behave appropriately in class and as a result enjoyed school more and stayed on track with his peer group.

Case 2. Wang Is Having Social Adjustment Problems during Her Freshman Year at College

Wang is an 18-year-old just beginning her college education at her state's flagship university, where she is studying civil engineering. She was a top student in her high school and particularly excelled in her math and science classes, making engineering a natural fit for her talents and interests. Winning a scholarship that covers her tuition and fees for four years at the state flagship sealed the deal, and she is eager to prove that she can handle the academic challenges that lie ahead.

Her parents, a physician and an electrical engineer, are proud of their daughter and have always encouraged her academic ambitions.

Wang is doing well in her first-semester courses, which include challenging required classes in calculus, physics, chemistry, and engineering design, but the classes are so large she feels she doesn't have a chance to get to know her professors or any of her fellow students. She's having more trouble finding her place within the social community of the university, which seems like a foreign world to her. Wang attended a Catholic, girls-only high school with a total of 600 students where she took part in many activities, including the robotics team, debate club, Model UN, and Scholastic Bowl, and also competed with the swim team and sang in the choir. All these activities kept her busy and provided ready-made friend groups without distracting from her studies. Wang felt that her high school was good: she worked hard and did well in her classes, which won her recognition at school and the approval of her parents, and she took part in a variety of activities with other students, all of which had low barriers to entry, so she never felt lonely.

The fact that Wang attended an all-girls school meant she was shielded from some of the issues young women in co-educational settings face, including how boys will react to their high achievements, particularly in fields culturally coded as male such as math and science. She didn't date in high school, largely due to the belief of her conservative parents that she should concentrate on her studies and that dating was not appropriate at her age. Things are very different at university, where there are over 30,000 students from diverse backgrounds, and where her fellow students in the engineering college are predominantly male. Activities that Wang enjoyed in high school seem to not exist in this new environment or are competitive and not open to all students. For instance, the swimming team consists primarily of recruited athletes on scholarship, while the debate club is competitive at the national level and everyone on the team competed at a higher level in high school than did Wang. She feels lonely and isolated, particularly when everyone around her seems to have already found their friend groups (many arrived with friends from their high school). Social expectations also are different from what she experienced in high school, and she's particularly confused by the dating scene: most students seem to have years of experience dating members of the opposite sex, and many are sexually active in what seems to Wang like a hookup culture that she doesn't want to be a part of.

Wang feels isolated and depressed, to the point where she seldom speaks to her fellow students, even before and after class. Uncertain of what is happening and losing confidence that she can succeed in her chosen career, Wang makes an appointment at the university counseling center. There, a counselor recognizes that she is experiencing culture shock due to the differences between her home and high school culture and that of the university culture in which she is now immersed. The counselor refers Wang to a staff psychologist, who diagnoses her as having ADHD, which is exacerbating her difficulty in adjusting to a new social environment. The psychologist explains that ADHD is a condition that can be treated, and Wang is relieved to hear that her difficulties are not the result of personal deficiencies or a failure to try hard enough. The psychologist suggests some books Wang could read that discuss ADHD from a woman's point of view and recommends that Wang set up a series of counseling appointments for the semester, during which she will learn behavioral techniques that will help her learn more about ADHD and practice interacting in social situations. She also recommends that Wang join some campus organizations that will help her meet like-minded people and provide her with a friend group, such as the Newman Society (an organization for Catholic students) and the student branch of Society of Women Engineers. She also emphasizes that people with ADHD often have trouble understanding social interactions but also emphasizes that Wang is entitled to make her own choices and should not feel compelled to conform to any aspect of university life which she feels goes against her personal values.

Analysis

Many students who were high achievers in high school find it difficult to adjust to university life, and sometimes the difficulties are more social and cultural than academic. Wang experienced greater culture shock than most, since she went from a small, all-girls, religiously affiliated school to a large, secular, co-ed state university. But she is determined to succeed and realized that she needed some help to make a successful adjustment to university life. The counselor recognized that there might be more than ordinary culture shock at work and referred Wang to a psychologist who evaluated her for ADHD. The psychologist determined that Wang met the diagnostic criteria for ADHD and recommended a combination of behavioral therapy and lifestyle modifications that would help Wang adjust to university life while maintaining her own values and identity.

Wang, who was eager to succeed in her studies and to find social relationships that worked for her, educated herself about ADHD, attended regular counseling sessions which helped her understand herself and learn effective ways to interact with people, and found several campus social organizations within which she felt at home. Joining the Newman Club (an organization for Catholic students) provided her with friends and adult mentors who shared her values and offered her with a "third place" on campus, separate from her classes and her dorm room, where she could go to relax. Joining the student chapter of the Society of Women Engineers allowed her to meet more women in her field and put her in touch with a female engineering faculty member who acted as an unofficial adviser to Wang throughout her undergraduate career.

Case 3. Juan Is Worried about Performing Well at His First Professional Job

Juan is 21 years old and recently graduated from university with a degree in business administration and a minor in finance. His parents both work in service jobs and are very proud of him, as he is the first member of his family to attend college. Juan interviewed with a number of companies during his senior year and has recently begun his first professional job as a market research analyst with a Fortune 500 company. He likes the job but also feels pressured to do well in his career so he can help his parents and younger siblings financially.

Everything went well at first, as new hires at this company begin their work experience with an extended orientation period during which they are introduced to the company and the different departments within it. However, real work has now begun and Juan is beginning to feel nervous about his ability to do the job. He is very eager to do well but is having trouble organizing his workload and is prone to making simple mistakes, which his supervisor attributes to carelessness and a failure to take the job seriously. Juan is concerned because the company treats the first year of employment as an extended apprenticeship, during which new hires receive quarterly reviews, and not every new hire is retained by the company. Given this structure, Juan's future with the company depends on his supervisor's recommendation that he be promoted to a permanent position at the end of his first year.

Confused about why he is struggling, and concerned that he might fail in his first professional job, Juan makes an appointment with a psychologist who specializes in adults experiencing workplace issues. After an interview, during which Juan explains his family, educational, and work history and the specific reasons why he made the appointment, the psychologist administers a number of tests and informs Juan that he has ADHD. Juan is taken aback at first, because he never considered that he might have some sort of mental or psychological impairment, but the psychologist explains that ADHD is not a disease but a condition, and that people with it have brains that work differently from what is considered "normal" in our society. More importantly, she assures him that people with ADHD can succeed in their careers, but they might need to make some adjustments to how they go about their work day.

The psychologist also informs Juan of his legal rights, but Juan does not want to disclose his diagnosis because he feels that he works in a competitive environment and it might hurt his chances to be retained were he to mention what they might consider a weakness, let alone ask for any accommodations. The psychologist assures him that it is entirely his choice whether to disclose or not, and that he can make changes to how he approaches his work that will help him succeed without identifying him as "a person with a disease." Juan's primary difficulties relate to distractibility and memory, so she suggests some simple measures that can help him with those issues without drawing attention to himself.

The office he works in uses an open plan and new hires do not have private offices, but there is a "quiet room" available for anyone to use. She suggests he be very mindful of the tasks he is assigned, and when he is doing work that requires particular concentration (e.g., calculations), he use the quiet room. She suggests that he take notice of when the office is most likely to be quiet and take advantage of those hours to do or check the work he is most concerned about. She also recommends keeping a notebook in which he can write down ideas that come to him without interrupting whatever he is currently doing, and that he use a paper planner in which he notes all upcoming deadlines and blocks out specific times during which he will do the work that requires the most concentration. She suggests he schedule regular check-ins with himself, on a daily, weekly, and monthly basis: at the start of each period, he will review what he needs to accomplish and schedule his time accordingly, while at the end of each period he will evaluate what he has completed and what remains to be done. She also recommends that he form the habit of breaking down every task into smaller subtasks, and noting those on his planner as well.

The psychologist assures him that many successful people use techniques like these to help them succeed at their jobs, and that they will not brand him as a person with a disability or as someone who is incapable of professional work. Quite the contrary: many executives use extensive systems of scheduling and self-examination to keep themselves working efficiently, and his employer will be impressed that he took the initiative to do so himself. She also asks him to spend time reviewing the ideas he jots down in his notebook, because they might contain important insights or ideas that could help set him apart from his fellow trainees.

Analysis

Juan's experience is typical of many people with ADHD who do well in the structured environment of university but experience difficulties in the more amorphous world of the workplace. Many adults with ADHD were not diagnosed as children and first become aware of their condition when it begins to cause them difficulties at work. Fortunately, Juan's symptoms are primarily those of executive function, and with the help of the psychologist he learned to manage them and receive good performance reviews in his trial year, as a result of which he was promoted to a permanent position with the company. Speaking with the psychologist also helped Juan's confidence, because he was starting to wonder if he was cut out for a professional job and tended to blame himself for the mistakes he made at work.

While helping him meet workplace expectations, the psychologist's suggestions also freed Juan up to capitalize on his creative powers. While previously his stray thoughts seemed only a distraction from completing his assigned work, when he formed the habit of writing them down and reviewing them later, he found he had some good suggestions for new ways the department could improve its functioning. His supervisor was impressed and some of his suggestions were put into place, as having the courage to think creatively and make suggestions in an appropriate and tactful manner impressed his supervisor and helped Juan stand out from among his peer group.

Case 4. Ashley Is Apprehensive about Taking a Drug Holiday

Ashley is 15 years old and looking forward to beginning her freshman year at a suburban high school in the coming fall. Two years ago, at age 13, her parents took her to a psychiatrist for an evaluation because she was struggling both academically and socially in her middle school. This was a new experience for Ashley, who had previously been a good if not excellent student and who got along well with her teachers and classmates. Her parents initially attributed Ashley's difficulties to changes in the school structure and atmosphere. In her grade school, she had one teacher for all subjects, and remained in the same classroom all day, so she got to know her classmates and teacher well. The school's leadership emphasized cooperation over competition and believed in bringing out the best in each student, whatever their talents might be, and there was no ranking or tracking of students. Her middle school was organized quite differently: students had a different teacher for each subject and moved from one classroom to another each period, a process which she found disruptive. Ashley found it difficult to get to know so many different classmates and teachers, and the coursework was also more difficult, which threatened her self-image as a good student. Students were assigned to specific classes in some subjects, such as math, based on their perceived aptitude, and grades were taken more seriously. With these changes, Ashley felt the spirit of cooperation from her grade school had been replaced by one of competition, and she felt inadequate to the task.

Ashley received a diagnosis of ADHD, inattentive type, and began taking Adderall and attending counseling sessions which helped her control her symptoms and better understand her condition. She learned a number of techniques that helped her succeed in her new school environment, and the combination of treatments was successful. Ashley became a solid "B" student with a talent for creative writing and had a solid group of friends, many of whom shared her interest in literature and writing.

Ashley is looking forward to high school, where she will have the chance to take more specialized courses in literature and foreign languages and where she will have more opportunities to develop her writing talents. She is particularly looking forward to writing for the school newspaper, joining the literary club, and taking part in the school's dramatics program. Her physician is impressed with how well she's doing on her treatment plan but is also mindful that there is some research evidence that taking stimulant medications such as Adderall over a period of years is associated with a lag in physical growth. She suggests Ashley take a drug holiday, during which time she would continue attending counseling sessions but would stop taking Adderall.

Ashley is concerned and upset and wonders why her psychiatrist would want to change a course of treatment that is working well for her. She was frustrated with her struggles in middle school, not understanding why her life suddenly seemed to have stopped working, and wants to continue taking the medication she feels gave her her life back. She's also concerned about making any major changes in treatment just as she will be entering a new period of adjustment, going from middle school to high school, and feels any changes to her treatment plan could jeopardize her ability to adjust successfully to the high school environment. She believes the competitive atmosphere she felt in middle school will be amped up in high school and that doing well in her classes is crucial to her plans to attend a good college and become a writer. She's also very concerned about making a good first impression on her teachers and her fellow students and feels that if she makes a bad beginning because her ADHD symptoms are interfering with her ability to function, they may write her off, limiting her possibilities for both academic achievement and friendships for her entire high school career.

The psychiatrist understands Ashley's worries and suggests that she take the drug holiday in the summer, a time when she will feel more relaxed and during which she has no important obligations. Her family has no major travel plans and Ashley is planning to spend the summer mostly hanging out with friends she already knows well, and who will be supportive should her ADHD symptoms get out of control. The psychiatrist explains to Ashley and her family that she would be carefully monitored during the drug holiday period, and that she could resume taking medication at any time if that seemed appropriate. She also reminds them that it might be good for Ashley's body to cease taking the drug for a period, and that it's also possible that Ashley no longer needs to take Adderall, since she's been doing so well with the behavioral techniques she has learned, but that they will never know unless she tries the drug holiday plan.

Analysis

Physicians are divided over the usefulness of drug holidays for ADHD patients, but many believe they can be a useful tool in specific circumstances. The fact that this drug holiday was suggested by the psychiatrist who has treated Ashley for two years and knows her well suggests that it may be an option worth trying (as opposed to a bad kind of drug holiday that is the result of a blanket policy and does not take individual differences into consideration). The psychiatrist was wise to suggest taking the drug holiday in the summer, rather than making any changes to a treatment plan just as the patient is entering a stressful period (such as beginning high school). The reasons are twofold: the stakes are higher if Ashley experiences a treatment failure during the school year, and it can be difficult to separate out any changes caused by the drug holiday from the changes caused by a new environment.

Ashley's physician did the right thing by stressing to her and her family that the drug holiday was a trial that could be ended at any time, and one during which she would be closely monitored. Framing the holiday as a treatment adjustment that could help Ashley, and during which she would be well-supported by her medical team, family, and friends, convinced Ashley and her parents to give it a try. She ceased taking Adderall for a period, but her symptoms returned to the point where the psychiatrist felt it was best that she resume taking it, although at a lower dose than before. Ashley felt the experience was worthwhile because she learned more about her condition and how it affected her functioning, and was stabilized on a lower dose of Adderall before beginning high school.

Case 5. Jordan's Parents Don't Believe ADHD Is Real

Jordan is African American and has been working at a local restaurant since graduating from high school two years ago. Now age 20, he wants to improve his job prospects by attending college, but his academic record is poor, due primarily to frequent absences and failure to complete assignments on time. Jordan feels he has the ability to succeed in college but doesn't know how to get started in the process. No one in his immediate family has attended college and he's not certain how the bureaucratic structures involved work. He's concerned about the costs of college, since his family cannot help with tuition, and doesn't know about the different types of financial aid for which he might be eligible.

Most of the students at the high school Jordan attended were white or Asian, and Jordan feels many teachers racially stereotyped him as a person who had no academic potential. As a result, he wasn't given the same feedback and attention other white students received, and his disinclination to meet academic expectations became a self-fulfilling prophecy. Even his guidance counselor didn't take his desire for further education seriously, and Jordan feels she regarded him as just another young Black man who didn't care about school. He spoke with a representative of a community organization that helps young adults who want to better their lives, and after hearing his story, a counselor at that organization recommended he see a psychologist to be evaluated for learning disabilities.

The psychologist diagnosed Jordan with ADHD and explained that this condition could help explain some of the difficulties he had experienced in formal education. She also told him that ADHD could be treated and controlled, so that it did not limit his ability to succeed in education or restrict his career choices. She referred him to a community center that provided low-cost counseling and suggested he be treated with behavioral therapy for ADHD. She also provided him with a referral to a different community organization that helps high school graduates apply for college and for financial aid. Jordan learned that, due to his income, he was eligible for the Pell Grant program, a type of federal financial aid that does not need to be repaid.

Jordan lives with his parents and three younger siblings. His parents, while supporting his ambition to attend college, reacted poorly to his news that he had been diagnosed with ADHD, which they regard as a "white folks' disease." At his next counseling session, Jordan asked his therapist if that statement was true, and if not, why his parents would believe it was. The therapist, an African American man, explained that it was true that many surveys have found that white people are more likely to receive an ADHD diagnosis, as compared to people of color (including Black, Hispanic, and Asian people). However, some surveys have found the opposite result, and in any case this discrepancy could be due to the underdiagnosis of nonwhite people rather than a real difference in the incidence of ADHD among racial and ethnic groups. He explained that in a country where people are not guaranteed access to health care, those with more money are likely to receive more and better care, including being able to meet with a psychiatrist or psychologist to be evaluated for ADHD. He also said that people in the medical and psychological communities are not immune to prejudice or misinformation, and that they could make the same mistake as his school counselor and ascribe behaviors typical of ADHD to cultural or personal factors, rather than evaluating a struggling student for ADHD.

Jordan made a series of weekly appointments to meet with a psychologist specializing in cognitive-behavioral therapy (CBT), a short-term and goal-oriented method of psychotherapy that has been shown to improve executive functioning and change the way a person thinks about themselves and their future. Jordan learned to recognize when he was engaging in counterproductive thinking and learned time-management skills that would help him break his pattern of procrastination and missed deadlines. The CBT sessions also helped him improve his self-image so that he began to see himself as someone who could succeed in higher education. As he learned more about ADHD, Jordan also felt more confident about speaking to his parents about it. Ultimately, he was able to convince them that ADHD did not occur only among white people, and that anyone who had ADHD could benefit from diagnosis and treatment. The community organization helped Jordan decide what he wanted out of college, helped him choose schools that would meet his needs, and helped him through the application and financial aid process. He decided to attend a local community college for two years and then apply to transfer to a four-year institution. This course of action meant he would not incur debt, as his Pell Grant was sufficient to cover his tuition and fees, and he could continue to work part-time at his current job and continue to live with his family.

Analysis

Unfortunately, stereotyping and prejudice are present at all levels of our society, even in fields like education and medicine. Also unfortunately, the procedures to apply for college and for financial aid in the United States are far from straightforward and may seem impossibly confusing to a first-generation student. Becoming aware of how prejudice and misinformation can shape the behavior of professionals can help someone who has been harmed by such behaviors, as can learning about different ways to overcome them. Jordan recognized that his high school record was not a fair indication of his academic abilities and refused to accept the judgment of his school teachers and counselors that he was simply not college material. Instead, he sought help from two community organizations to learn more about himself and find out what he could do to achieve the life that he wanted.

After receiving a diagnosis of ADHD from a psychologist, Jordan took part in a series of CBT appointments which helped him recognize counterproductive behavior patterns he had previously engaged in and to substitute new behaviors that would help him succeed. These appointments also helped Jordan learn about ADHD, so that he was able to speak to his parents about it, eventually overcoming convincing them that it was a real condition that could affect people of any race or ethnicity. Jordan worked with a second community organization to clarify his goals for higher education, then to apply for and be accepted to a program that set him on a path to achieve his goals.

Glossary

Accommodations: Changes made in an environment to meet the needs of an individual, for instance, changes in the school environment for a student diagnosed with ADHD. Examples of common accommodations for ADHD include extra time on exams, the use of technology to help the student stay organized, break times throughout the classroom day, and provision of written materials to accompany lectures.

ADD: Attention Deficit Disorder, a term that has been replaced by ADHD (Attention Deficit/Hyperactivity Disorder) in professional discourse, although the term ADD may still be seen in older publications.

ADHD: Attention Deficit Hyperactivity Disorder, the modern term for a disorder defined in *DSM-5-TR* as being characterized by behaviors such as inattention, hyperactivity, and impulsiveness. Note that "ADHD" is commonly used to refer to this condition even if hyperactivity is not present in an individual patient.

Americans with Disability Act (ADA): A 1990 federal law that recognizes ADHD as a disability, and allows people with ADHD to request appropriate accommodations so they may do their job.

Attentional bias: The tendency of people to focus on some things while ignoring others. Attentional bias is normal, and everyone displays it from time to time, because in order to concentrate on one thing, you must ignore others. For instance, if you are studying with great concentration, you may not notice when someone else comes into the room. Attentional bias is only a problem for people with ADHD if it interferes with their functioning, for instance, if they regularly miss social cues that other people notice easily.

Behavioral training: A type of therapy often used to help adolescents and adults with ADHD. The purpose of the training is to make the individual more conscious of what situations cause them difficulties and to practice positive behaviors that will help them succeed.

CDC: The Centers for Disease Control and Prevention, a federal agency in the United States that funds, promotes, and disseminates research and information about public health topics, including ADHD. The CDC website includes links to many datasets collected by different federal agencies and many publications by those agencies.

CHADD: Children and Adults with Attention-Deficit/Hyperactivity Disorder, a national organization founded in 1987 in the United States to provide support, education, and advocacy for people with ADHD, their families, and caregivers. CHADD operates the National Resource Center on ADHD (NRC), a clearinghouse for evidence-based information about ADHD, and receives funding from the

Centers for Disease Control and Prevention and the National Center on Birth Defects and Developmental Disabilities.

Cognitive flexibility: The ability of a person to switch their mind between one topic or task and another when it is appropriate to do so. Cognitive flexibility is key in many problem-solving situations, where a person needs to be able to change from an approach that isn't working to one that might. People with ADHD are sometimes deficient in cognitive flexibility, which can be a problem in school and work situations where they are expected to shift their attention as directed.

Combined type: One of the three subtypes of ADHD in which a person experiences both inattentive and hyperactive symptoms.

Complementary and alternative medicine (CAM): Treatments outside the range of standard Western medicine, such as yoga, acupuncture, and nutritional supplements. While research into the effectiveness of CAM for ADHD is still in its early stages, some people have found that CAM treatments are helpful in managing their symptoms, and many physicians are open to the idea of including CAM alongside more conventional medical treatments.

Co-existing conditions: A term similar in meaning to "comorbidities" with regard to medical conditions. Coexisting conditions means that one individual is affected by several different conditions at the same time (for instance, a person has both ADHD and depression).

DSM-5-TR: *The Diagnostic and Statistical Manual of Mental Disorders*, 5th edition, text revision, the most recent version of the handbook published by the American Psychiatric Association which is the authoritative guide used in the United States and in some other countries to diagnose mental health disorders, including ADHD.

Executive function: A set of skills that allow an individual to control and coordinate their cognitive abilities and behaviors, for instance, to plan, coordinate, and carry out tasks to meet goals which may require some time to complete. People with ADHD often struggle with executive function, but it can be improved with practice and the use of external aids (e.g., planners and automated reminder systems), and good executive functioning plays an important role in many aspects of adult life.

Externalizing disorders: Conditions like oppositional defiant disorder (ODD) and conduct disorder (CD) that are characterized by a lack of cooperation and defiance toward authority figures (ODD), and a general disregard for rules and socially acceptable behavior. Both disorders occur more commonly in children with ADHD than in the general population, and more commonly in boys than girls, but are distinct disorders from ADHD and should be recognized as coexisting conditions.

FAPE: Free and Appropriate Public Education, a right established under Section 504 of the Rehabilitation Act of 1973 and the Individuals with Disabilities Education Act. The idea behind FAPE is that every child is entitled to a free public education that meets their needs, and that it is the responsibility of local school districts to provide that education, including any necessary evaluation of the student and a customized educational plan if necessary.

Hyperfocus: A state in which a person is completely absorbed in a task to the exclusion of noticing anything else. Hyperfocus can be a strength, because many breakthroughs in research only occur after long and sustained concentration, but it can also be a problem in school and at work if a person is reluctant or unable to shift their attention when directed to do so.

ICD-10: The International Classification of Diseases, Tenth Revision, is the most recent version of the classification system for disease created and published by the World Health Organization. The ICD-10 includes diagnosis codes used by physicians to classify diagnoses, symptoms, and procedures, and are used in claims systems, for data collection and research, health care administration and service planning.

Individuals with Disabilities Education Act: A 1990 federal law that requires school districts to meet the educational needs of each student, including granting appropriate accommodations, providing necessary technology, and paying for the student to receive services elsewhere if the school district cannot provide them.

Inhibition control: The ability to manage and control one's thoughts, emotions, and behaviors. What is appropriate depends on the context and age of the individual, and most people learn inhibition control as they mature, but people with ADHD may struggle with it.

Learning disorders: Conditions that make it difficult for a student to learn. Symptoms of learning disorders include reversing letters and numbers (after second grade), difficulty with manual tasks such as writing, and difficulty in recognizing patterns and sorting items by size and shape. The three major types of learning disorders are dyslexia (difficulty with reading), dyscalculia (difficulty with math), and dysgraphic (difficulty with writing), and any or all of these may occur alongside ADHD.

Medication holiday: Also called a drug holiday, a period of time during which a person who normally takes one or more prescribed medications temporarily discontinues them. Medication holidays are planned in conjunction with medical advice and should be monitored to see how the individual reacts when they stop taking their medications, and to intervene if necessary.

Mental Health and Addiction Equality Act of 2008: A federal law that requires most health insurance plans to cover mental health and substance use disorders on a parity basis with medical conditions.

MRI: Magnetic Resonance Imaging, a type of noninvasive medical technology that allows researchers to study which brain areas are activated in people with and without ADHD under particular conditions.

Parent behavioral therapy training: a treatment method often recommended for parents of children younger than 12 with ADHD, in which the child's parents are taught skills and strategies to help their child control their symptoms and succeed in school and in relationships. Parental behavioral therapy is generally taught over a number of sessions (often 8–12), with the understanding that the parents will practice whatever they are learning (for instance, effective use of positive reinforcement) with their child between sessions.

Pomodoro technique: A method of studying which some people with ADHD (also many without ADHD) find effective. In this technique, the student uses a timer to study for a predetermined amount of time (often 20 or 25 minutes), followed by a short break (often 5 minutes), and then the cycle is repeated. This technique promotes retention of material by alternating periods of focused study interspersed with rest periods.

Primarily hyperactive: One of the three subtypes of ADHD, a person with a primarily hyperactive diagnosis experiences challenges such as constant fidgeting, being unable to work quietly, talking excessively and speaking out of turn, and being unable to remain seated in a classroom. As the name suggests, these behaviors have in common an excess ("hyper-") of activity level given what is socially appropriate in a situation.

Primarily inattentive: One of the three subtypes of ADHD. A person with a primarily inattentive diagnosis tends to experience issues such as making careless mistakes, failing to follow clear directions, losing concentration in the midst of a task, or regularly failing to complete work they have previously committed to.

Rebound effect: A situation sometimes experienced when a person stops taking a prescribed medication due to which their symptoms come back worse than before they started taking the medication. The possibility of a rebound effect is one reason medication holidays should be planned and supervised by a medical professional.

Section 504: A section of the Rehabilitation Act of 1973 which specifies the rights of students with ADHD and the legal responsibilities of the school district toward them. The rights include a no-cost evaluation and appropriate educational services to meet the students' needs.

Social Skills Training (SST): A type of counseling and coaching intended to help clients understand and practice the norms of social interaction, such as taking turns in conversation or communicating appropriately with coworkers in an office.

Subthreshold ADHD: A condition in which a person has some of the symptoms of ADHD, but their symptoms are not sufficient to receive a clinical diagnosis. As diagnosis is not an exact science, and a person with subthreshold ADHD may experience symptoms that interfere with their functioning, they may well benefit from interventions similar to those for someone with clinically diagnosed ADHD.

Therapeutic use exemption (TUE): An official decision, made by a governing body in a sport such as the NCAA (US colleges) or WADA (international competition), allowing an individual to use a prescribed medication which is otherwise banned. Some drugs used to treat ADHD are stimulants which are classified as banned substances, but an individual who is prescribed those drugs to treat their ADHD can apply for a therapeutic use exemption to be able to take the drug while competing in their chosen sport.

Working memory: Information a person holds in the front of their mind while completing a task, such as remembering a phone number long enough to dial it. People with ADHD often have deficiencies in their working memory and may exhibit behaviors such as needing to constantly reread directions or to recall basic information when needed.

Directory of Resources

Apps

MyHomework: https://myhomeworkapp.com A cross-platform planner application designed specifically for students in junior high and older to help keep track of assignments and deadlines; it includes the ability to prioritize tasks, receive reminders of upcoming deadlines, and mark tasks as completed.

Pomofocus: https://pomofocus.io/ A customizable web-based application that facilitates using the pomodoro time-management technique, and produces reports of time spent on different tasks.

RescueTime: https://www.rescuetime.com/ A web-based application that works in the background to track user activity and create reports, which gives users an accurate picture of how they are actually spending their time online; the premium version includes the ability to limit time spent on specified websites.

TickTick: https://ticktick.com/ A cross-platform planner application that allows users to keep track of recurring tasks and create customized to-do lists with priorities and due dates. The app also displays deadlines on a calendar and sends reminders to the user as completion dates near.

Books

Barkley, Russell. *Managing ADHD in School: The Best Evidence-Based Methods for Teachers*. Eu Claire, WI: PESI Publishing & Media, 2016. A guidebook to ADHD written by a psychologist for K–12 educators that provides an overview of the condition and research-based suggestions about how to help students with ADHD.

Guare, Richard, Dawson, Peg, and Guare, Colin. *Smart but Scattered Teens: The Revolutionary "Executive Skills" Approach to Helping Teens Reach Their Potential*. New York: Guilford Press, 2012. A self-help book for parents of teenagers who struggle with executive skills, based on scientific research and written by two psychologists and a young adult who worked through similar issues himself.

Levrini, Abigail L. *Succeeding with Adult ADHD: Daily Strategies to Help You Achieve Your Goals*. 2nd ed. Washington, DC: American Psychological Association, 2023. A guide for adults who have, or suspect they have, ADHD, which explains the condition and available treatments and provides suggestions and strategies for success in many aspects of life, including planning, social relationships, study skills, employment, and time management.

Miller, Kelli. *Thriving with ADHD Workbook for Kids*. Ill. by Sarah Rebar. New York: Althea Press, 2018. Written by a licensed clinical social worker for children ages 7–12 (with an introduction for parents), this book includes information and activities designed to help children with ADHD understand themselves and their condition and develop skills to help them succeed.

Millichap, J. Gordon. *Attention Deficit Hyperactivity Disorder Handbook: A Physician's Guide to ADHD*. 2nd ed. New York: Springer, 2013. A summary of what is known about ADHD and related disorders, with extensive references to the medical literature, this book will be useful to more advanced students who want an in-depth overview of the condition, particularly if they are considering a career in medicine or scientific research.

Quinn, Patricia O. *Attention, Girls! A Guide to Learn All about Your AD/HD*. Washington, DC: American Psychological Association, 2021. Written by a pediatrician, this illustrated self-help guide is written for girls in junior high and high school to help them understand ADHD and use effective strategies to cope with their symptoms.

Saline, Sharon. *What Your ADHD Child Wishes You Knew: Working Together to Empower Kids for Success in School and Life*. New York: TarcherPerigee, 2018. A practical guide for parents of children ages 6–18 who have ADHD which explains the condition in layman's terms and offers advice and exercises to help children with ADHD succeed.

Wolraich, Mark L., and Hagan, Joseph F. *ADHD: What Every Parent Needs to Know*. 3rd ed. Itasca, IL: American Academy of Pediatrics, 2019. Written by two physicians, this book provides information about ADHD and advice for parents of children diagnosed with ADHD, from early childhood through the teen years.

Organizations

ADDitude: https://www.additudemag.com. An online community for people with ADHD which publishes an online magazine for laymen and maintains a variety of information about ADHD on its web page. There is a fee for subscribing to the magazine, which is available in both print and digital forms, but other information is available for free from the website. Much of the information on the website is written by professionals, but user content is also available (e.g., medication reviews) and there is a strong focus on self-help and sharing strategies among people with ADHD and their families.

The Attention Deficit Disorder Association (ADDA): https://add.org. A 501-C2 nonprofit organization of adults with ADHD whose purpose is to help their members thrive. Membership includes access to an online community with many support groups for specific types of individuals (e.g., for women over 50, for partners of adults with ADHD, for African Americans) and with particular focuses (e.g., productivity, accountability at work). Basic information about ADHD is available on the organization's website, as is a professional referral directory, but the primary focus is to facilitate adults with ADHD sharing experiences and helping each other.

CHADD (Children and Adults with Attention Deficit/Hyperactivity Disorder): https://chadd.org. An organization founded in 1987 with the goal to improve the lives of people with ADHD. It has chapters throughout the United States. CHADD maintains a website which contains basic information about ADHD and a directory of resources, and it regularly hosts conferences and training events, and hosts the National Resource Center on ADHD.

Professional Organizations

The American Academy for Child and Adolescent Psychiatry: https://www.aacap. org. A professional medical organization whose membership includes 10,000 child and adolescent psychiatrists, both in the United States and abroad, plus some members who are students or physicians specializing in other fields. They maintain an online resource center which provides resources to clinicians and also provides basic information about ADHD in laymen's terms for people with ADHD, their caregivers, and educators.

The American Academy of Pediatrics: https://www.aap.org/en/ and www. healthychildren.org. A professional medical association of physicians specializing in the treatment of infants, children, adolescents, and young adults. The APA regularly issues policy statements on relevant subjects, advocates for child health, and offers a number of opportunities for physicians to share knowledge and further their education. The first website includes information about ADHD for professionals, while the second site focuses on providing information to parents.

The American Psychological Association: https://www.apa.org. A professional organization for people holding a doctoral degree in psychology, with associate and affiliate memberships available to students, teachers at the high school and community college level, and those holding a master's degree in psychology. They maintain an online resource page having information about ADHD, with both continuing education materials for professionals and materials written at a laymen's level, including articles, videos, and podcasts.

The Centers for Disease Control and Prevention (CDC): https://www.cdc.gov. A federally funded agency in the United States that funds research, provides services, and disseminates information about public health. It is a reliable source of information which collects and provides access to many datasets and information sources on health matters, and maintains a web page with information about ADHD for both health care professionals and the general public.

The Council of Parent Attorneys and Advocates (COPAA): https://www.copaa.org/default.aspx. A peer-to-peer network of attorneys, advocates, related professionals, and parents whose goal is to protect and enforce the legal and civil rights of students with disabilities. Their website includes a searchable database of attorneys, advocates, and other professionals (by geographic area and specialty), information about the rights of children with disabilities, a discussion board, and educational materials.

The Special Needs Alliance: https://www.specialneedsalliance.org. A national alliance of attorneys who provide services to individuals with disabilities and their families, including people with ADHD who are seeking accommodations in the workplace or feel they have been discriminated against. Their website includes a searchable directory of attorneys and an information center with information about legal issues relevant to people with disabilities.

Websites

ADHD/LD Resources: https://learningcenter.unc.edu/tips-and-tools/resources-and-tips-for-students-with-adhdld/ A website maintained by the University of North Carolina at Chapel Hill containing information and resources intended to help college students with ADHD understand their condition and succeed in their studies.

American Academy of Pediatrics: Supporting Students with Attention Deficit/Hyperactivity Disorder (ADHD) in Schools: https://www.aap.org/en/patient-care/school-health/mental-health-in-schools/supporting-students-with-attention-deficithyperactivity-disorder-adhd-in-schools/ A website run by a professional association for pediatricians which offers links to resources, reports, and policy statement helpful to physicians who advocate for children and adolescents with ADHD.

Attention-Deficit Hyperactivity Disorder (ADHD): https://www.cdc.gov/ncbddd/adhd/data.html. A website maintained by the Centers for Disease Control and Prevention providing easy access to information about ADHD, including basic information for laymen, facts and statistics, recent research, and written and audiovisual educational materials.

Attention-Deficit/Hyperactivity Disorder (ADHD): https://www.nimh.nih.gov/health/topics/attention-deficit-hyperactivity-disorder-adhd. A website maintained by the National Institute of Mental Health providing basic information about ADHD, footnoted with research sources and notes about the national surveys from which some of the statistical information was drawn.

Benefits.Gov: Your Path to Government Benefits (ADHD Resources): https://www.benefits.gov/news/article/471. A website created by the federal government to inform people about benefits to which they may be entitled, and to help them access those benefits.

CHADD: The National Resource Center: https://chadd.org/about/about-nrc/. A clearinghouse for expert-vetted, evidence-based information about ADHD, managed by CHADD in conjunction with the Centers for Disease Control and Prevention and the National Center for Birth Defects and Developmental Disabilities, it contains information for professionals, parents, and people with ADHD.

Know Your Rights: Students with ADHD: https://www2.ed.gov/about/offices/list/ocr/docs/dcl-know-rights-201607-504.pdf. Information from the United States Department of Education about the rights of students with ADHD, with links to resources and instructions about how to file a complaint if a student's needs are not being met.

Reddit ADHD Forum: https://www.reddit.com/r/ADHD/ An online forum about ADHD which also serves as a community to discuss ADHD, which also serves as an online community for people with ADHD. There are also specific forums within the Reddit website for different groups within the ADHD community, including adults with ADHD, people with ADHD who are on the autism spectrum, parents of children with ADHD, computer programmers with ADHD, and so on. While these forums (also called subreddits) can be useful sources of information, anything posted on them should be evaluated with care, because they are not professionally vetted.

Index

About the Author

Sarah Boslaugh is a Professional Tutor in Mathematics and Economics in the St. Louis Community College System. Prior to taking that position, she worked as a research analyst and statistician for twenty years, at employers including the New York City Public Schools, Montefiore Medical Center (New York City), the Washington University School of Medicine (Saint Louis, Missouri), and BJC HealthCare (Saint Louis, Missouri). She received her Ph.D. in Measurement and Evaluation from the City University of New York and her MPH from Saint Louis University. Her previous books include *An Intermediate Guide to SPSS Programming, Statistics in a Nutshell, Secondary Data Sources for Public Health: A Practical Guide,* and *Transgender Health Issues.*